ENDORSEMENTS

Doc Shannan helped me stay in top physical form while on the ATP tour. His book, *The Original Design for Health*, can help you achieve & maintain optimal health, too!

Andy Roddick
Former World #1 Professional Tennis Player
"Fastest Serve in a Grand Slam" Record Holder
Founder of the Andy Roddick Foundation to help at-risk youth

This book is a "must-read" for anyone who's trying to achieve a higher level of health potential. After helping so many, Dr. Mark has put this method in a simple and practical way for you to start implementing immediately. It's time that you discover *your* Original Design for health! Remember, your health is your best investment!

Dr. Fab Mancini
"Healthy Living" Media Expert
International Best-selling Author and Speaker

THE
ORIGINAL
DESIGN
FOR
HEALTH

THE
ORIGINAL
DESIGN
FOR
HEALTH

THE **SIMPLE PLAN** TO
RESTORE & MAINTAIN
HEALTH IN **3 EASY STEPS**

DR. MARK SHANNAN

DESTINY IMAGE® PUBLISHERS, INC.

P.O. Box 310, Shippensburg, PA 17257-0310

"Promoting Inspired Lives."

This book and all other Destiny Image and Destiny Image Fiction books are available at Christian bookstores and distributors worldwide.

Interior design by Susan Ramundo

Jacket design by Eileen Rockwell

Author photo by Korey Howell (koreyhowellphotography.com)

Hair stylist: Anh Hoang Nguyen

Graphic art designs by Gabrielle Shannan

For more information on foreign distributors, call 717-532-3040.

Reach us on the Internet: www.destinyimage.com.

ISBN 13 TP: 978-0-7684-0987-1

ISBN 13 eBook: 978-0-7684-0953-6

ISBN 13 HC: 978-0-7684-0952-9

For Worldwide Distribution, Printed in the U.S.A.

1 2 3 4 5 6 7 8 / 20 19 18 17 16

DISCLAIMER

The sole purpose of this book is to provide general health information based on research and years of clinical and life experience. This information is not intended for use in the diagnosis, prevention, or cure of any disease. If you have any serious, acute, or chronic health concerns, please consult a trained health professional who can fully assess your needs and address them effectively. Dr. Shannan cannot give any advice, treatment, or counsel to any readers of this book unless they're already an established patient and are currently under his care for the condition in question.

DEDICATION

If you sit and think about it, all of us have one person in our lives who, we can say with a great degree of certainty, has been our greatest influence and mentor. My father, Dr. George Martin Shannan, is a doctor of chiropractic and a clinical nutritionist who's been in constant practice for over 56 years, and he's still practicing today. He is *that* person in my life.

Through the years, I've learned from his example of love, expertise in chiropractic, exercise, faith, nutritional guidance, financial wisdom, grace and devotion toward others, gentleness of spirit, and a desire to help those in need. His legacy of having a heart focused on God, health, family, and helping others will hopefully live on through me and my children, and their children too. I've always looked up to him, admired him, and always wanted to be "just like my dad."

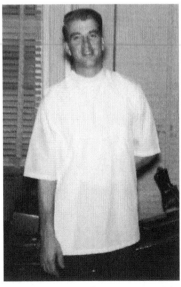

Therefore, I dedicate this book to him with a heart that's full and a debt of gratitude that I'll never be able to repay. You are the very definition of a good man, the best friend a guy could have, and you're my hero. I love you, Dad!

(His first year of practice, 1960)

ACKNOWLEDGMENTS

There are so many people I'd like to thank who've been a part of the journey of writing this book. First and foremost, I have to thank the one true God almighty, the Master Designer of all things, who gives me every breath that I take and every beat of my heart, and who gave me the inspiration for this book, and with whom all things are possible.

I'd like to thank my beautiful wife, Gabrielle, who loves me with the deepest kind of love, has always believed in me, accepts me as I am, and supports me in all that I do, even creating the graphic art for this book. She's my best friend, my biggest fan, and has always pointed me back to God when times have been tough. Thank you, love. To my girls, Audrey and Katie, who inspire me to be the best dad I can be, who love me with purity of heart and constantly remind me of the amazing joy and beauty that this life has to offer.

I'd like to thank my mom and dad who have always been there for me, taught me the morals and values that I operate by every day of my life, and who are the examples of parenthood and marriage that every child needs and dreams of. My mom always taught me to be my own person and how important it is to be loving, selfless, gentle, and kind. I've truly been blessed to not only have them as parents but as the best of friends.

I'd like to give an especially huge thanks to my brother-in-law, Pastor Rob Koke, and sister, Dr. Laura Koke, who have also been huge influences and examples of faith, balance, health, and what marriage should look like. Without their love, support, and guidance I wouldn't have been shaped into the man that I am today, and this book would not have been possible. Also, to my sister Gayle, who, since I was little, loved me, included her little brother in whatever she did, taught me how to be cool, and has always encouraged me.

In addition, I want to thank all of the people whose support, belief in this project, advice, guidance, and willingness to help me through the process of publishing a book have been absolutely priceless and will forever be appreciated: Dr. Jordan Rubin, Ronda Ranalli, Pastor Joel Osteen, Shannon Marven, Nan Hazel, Allen Arnold, Dr. Fab Mancini, and Andy Roddick.

CONTENTS

PILLAR III: CHEMICAL

PILLAR IV: SPIRITUAL

CONCLUSION

FOREWORD

Let me pose a question to you: Do you believe that God designed this universe and everything in it? If you answered yes to that question, then you probably also believe that God designed *you* and a way for you to live a healthy life. That would mean that He planned out every aspect of your life in such a way that achieving your full health potential could be simple and straightforward. Why would He want to make something that's so important be difficult and confusing? He wouldn't and He didn't. You can absolutely reach your body's fullest potential for health with a very simple plan…here's how I know.

My story: I was raised in a family with a dad who was a chiropractor and naturopathic physician, and a loving mother who prepared healthy meals that didn't consist of the standard junk foods common in the standard American diet. I understood many principles of living a healthy lifestyle, but I didn't continue living by those principles in college. I began to severely shift my diet over to processed foods that my body could not handle. It wasn't designed to handle them. I also began to get out of balance in several other important ways, like stress and sleep.

At the age of 19, I was so ill with severe Crohn's disease, in addition to a list of nearly 20 other ailments, that I was emaciated and within a breath of dying. I had tried every kind of medical treatment in the hospitals that doctors knew to prescribe. I had tried every supplement, herb, and "natural" diet known to man. I had visited with all of the health experts of the day and traveled to alternative treatment facilities all over the world. Nothing worked until…

When it seemed that all was lost, I began to simply eat the foods that God designed for us to eat. I avoided all of the processed, engineered "techno-foods" that humans had created using chemicals and processes that severely alter food from the Original Design. During a 40-day health experience I later deemed The Maker's Diet, my body began to transform and function the way that it was designed to. I had discovered that what I needed had been available all along—from the beginning of time.

Once my health was restored I was filled with a passion, a mission, and a clear purpose to help transform the health of God's people one life at a time. I continued my studies in health and nutrition, and it became clear to me that there were other components to living a healthy life that simply could not be ignored. After years of education and training and conversations with health professionals and spiritual leaders worldwide, I came to the realization that one achieved optimal health and wholeness in body, mind, soul, and spirit. Of course, God had an Original Design for those as well.

Dr. Mark Shannan is a friend and fellow natural-health crusader who also has an amazing passion for helping others restore and maintain the kind of health that God designed us all to live with. We share this passion for changing the world and seeing the sick and hurting restored to health. I am thrilled to be on the same team with someone as caring, compassionate, and rooted in God's design for health as Dr. Mark is. We've both found that understanding the basic foundational principles to health is the critical first step to achieving the vital health we all yearn for. In knowledge is the power to change.

This book is filled with information and insight that can absolutely turn your health challenges around and turn them into victories! Dr. Mark's heart to help others is evident in all that he does and he shares it in such a relatable and easy-to-understand way that you'll have trouble putting *The Original Design for Health* down.

The wisdom, information, and simple plan he's packed into this book is truly life changing. If you follow it, you'll never be the same. If you look to *the* Original Designer, you'll find all of the answers that you've been searching for. A new, healthier you awaits!

Jordan Rubin, NMD, PhD
New York Times bestselling author: *The Maker's Diet*
Founder: Garden of Life, Beyond Organic
Founder and CEO: Get Real Nutrition

INTRODUCTION

Howdy! In Texas we always make introductions, so let me introduce myself. My name is Dr. Mark Shannan. I'm a second-generation doctor of chiropractic and a clinical nutritionist born and raised in Austin, Texas. This book is the culmination of over 40 years of life's journey, school training, postgraduate courses, clinical experience, and wisdom imparted to me by dozens of brilliant men and women whose seminars, sermons, books, and conversations have shaped me into who I am today.

I wrote this book because every time I work with a patient or pray with a friend or hear of someone who relates their lack of peace, pain, or general unhealthiness, it makes my heart hurt for them. At the very same time, it makes me want to jump into their struggle, alongside them, and help guide them toward the kind of health that they deserve—optimal health based on the Original Design.

I've always been like this. I can't help it. It's how I was *designed*. I have a framed, two-line piece of homework from second grade in my office that reads, "When I grow up I will be a doctr cuz I like to help peopl." Thanks for saving it, Mom!

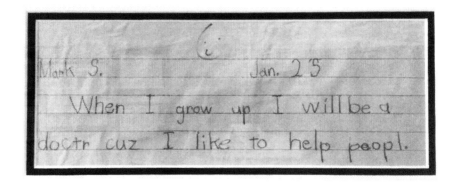

My handwriting has gotten considerably worse, but my spelling has changed for the better since those days. The one thing that hasn't changed, though, is my heart and my purpose. I still like to help people. In fact, I love it! I trust that God has a reason for causing my heart to beat fast as I think about the health of the people of this world. I am routinely awakened in the middle of the night with just a few simple thoughts or occasionally even large sections of information to impart that I know can touch people's lives.

I believe I've been given this information, a passion to help others and a vision for this book for one simple purpose: to help people live the most balanced, peace-filled, and healthy lives possible, the way they were intended, according to the Original Design.

WHAT'S GOING ON?

Okay, so here's the deal…the health of the people in industrialized nations, especially the United States, is in an extremely dangerous downward spiral. We're getting sicker and sicker. Despite amazing advancements in science, medicine, and technology, and despite having the best hospitals and doctors in the world, we're taking more medications, getting more vaccinations, and seeing the rates of serious diseases like heart disease, obesity, autism, diabetes, and cancer skyrocket. How we're living just isn't working.

The leading cause of death in America is still cardiovascular disease, with over 611,000 people per year, and cancer is #2 with more than 584,000 deaths per year.[1] A total of 225,000 deaths are attributed to medical treatment of some kind, which currently makes it the third leading cause of death in America.[2]

Sadly, 69% of adults aged 20 years and over in the US are overweight and 35.1% are obese.[3] One in five children has adult onset (type 2) diabetes. We have reduced the human sperm count by over 50% in the last 50 years, and it's still dropping.[4] Fertility clinics are popping up all over the place as more than 15% of all couples can't seem to get pregnant.[5] The truth is, we're on a very scary pace toward the extinction of our own species!

Over 106,000 people die every year from non-error, adverse effects of medication,[6] which means it wasn't the wrong medication or too much of it, but that the person's body simply couldn't handle it and they died. What is going on? "How could this be?" you may be asking. I'd suggest that it's for many different reasons—all of them, though, are evidence of a departure from the Original Design.

Chew on this for a minute: If traditional cultures that still live out in "the jungle" and adhere to their traditional diets and lifestyles are *not* getting these diseases and issues at anywhere near the rates that we are, then there has clearly got to be something that we're doing that they aren't. They're still doing what they've done for thousands of years, which has allowed their populations and way of living to continue the way they always have. (Granted, there are hardly any of these cultures left.)

You might be saying to yourself, "The people in those traditional cultures didn't live very long either." You'd be partially right if you're talking about the fact that many of them died due to infectious diseases after "modern" man showed up. However, there are several documented cultures, untouched by modern humans, that did routinely have individuals live to be over 100. We're not dying of infectious diseases, though; we're dying of chronic diseases of lifestyle like diabetes, obesity, cardiovascular disease, and cancer.

"Civilized" or "modern" humans are being exposed to and consuming chemicals, toxins, engineered "foods," and genetically modified organisms (GMOs) that have *never existed* prior to this century. We're creating more and more of these unnatural substances and taking them into our bodies at astounding and ever-increasing rates.

It's been estimated that over 10,000 chemical additives are allowed in our food by the FDA, and there are close to 100,000 registered chemicals/drugs in the books that are used in everything from our foods to medicine and industry. We're exposed to many if not most of these chemicals in our environment in some shape or form. And the vast majority of these chemicals weren't even in existence 100 years ago.

Additionally, our intake of processed sugar has increased from around six pounds per person per year in the 1800s to over 100 pounds per person per year in the 2000s—that's an 1,800% increase! In general, people in the US are eating nearly *double* the amount of calories that we need to live and thrive, and we have the most obese people of any developed nation.

We've become increasingly lazy and sedentary, spending very little time exercising or being active as we spend more time staring at computers or other electronic devices. We've become accustomed to and expect a high level of convenience because we don't want to work too hard or "get our hands dirty."

We're filling our minds with polluted thinking, pop psychology, mindless trash on TV, opinions of people who don't really know what they're talking about, and following counterfeit cultural fads that lead us astray. Our stress levels are at all-time highs which devastates our health in so many ways that it's virtually incalculable.

Our spirits are being filled with empty and false ideologies that have no foundation on the Master Designer of us all and everything in our world… the one true God. We've begun to "worship self" and to overvalue things, status, people, and power. We've lost sight of anything greater than just ourselves.

We're now several generations of people who've been educated, or more like "brainwashed," by marketers on TV, radio, the Internet, and print, who seek to train us to buy whatever product it is that they've been paid to sell. We're finding out every day through research that we're essentially the guinea pigs of some crazy chemical experiments that are killing us. We are living crash test dummies who are losing our lives as we find out what happens when we begin to alter what was originally designed to work so well.

For prescription medications alone, more than $11 billion is spent each year by pharmaceutical companies solely on promotion and marketing, $5 billion of which goes to sales representatives. "It's been estimated that $8,000 to $13,000 is spent per year on each physician." This is about $30 million each day.[7] Do you think they're more concerned with you getting a good education in how to stay healthy naturally or selling their drugs? Yep, exactly. Can anyone think of a better use of $11 billion for the health of humans? I sure can.

We've begun to veer so far from what we were designed to do and who we were designed to be that we're creating a life that's nearly devoid of health. We've truly lost focus. We're getting sicker by the minute and dying before our time, by the hundreds of thousands every year! The further we've gotten away from the Original Design, the bigger our problems have become, both personally and collectively.

THAT'S "MY BAD"

Additionally, so many people have stopped taking responsibility for their own health. They're simply doing whatever feels good and whatever they want to do without any thought for what'll happen to them in the future. After things are a complete mess, and their health is failing them, they're looking to our health-care system to fix the problems that *they* have mostly created.

So often I'll be talking with a patient, who's in a great deal of pain, and asks, "What can *you* do to fix me?" Only occasionally do I hear, "What can I do to fix this?" Those questions are extremely different. One wants an instant fix that they don't have to do anything for, and the other recognizes their need to take responsibility for their own health and be a larger part of the solution.

Have you ever heard someone on a sports team say, "My bad!" after they make a mistake? They simply take responsibility for messing up, and the whole team keeps going. When we deny the fact that we're the ones making poor choices that adversely affect our health, as well as those around us, everyone suffers. We're in denial about our poor health being directly related to our decisions, which makes it really hard to change. It's important for us to stop blaming others, look in the mirror, and refer to the Original Design to restore health.

We have a time during the service of our church where people can come up to the front and join hands in prayer with other members. I've prayed with a lot people who are well-meaning when they want to pray for God to heal their problems. However, many of them are unwilling to make any changes themselves. Prayer is extremely important in my opinion, but there's another step…

I've way too frequently heard something like, "I'd like to pray that God heals me of my diabetes, obesity, and cardiovascular disease. I just don't understand why this has to happen to me." While there are certainly health issues that are beyond our control, many of them, if not most of them, are products of our choices and our lifestyles. We have to be willing to do our part in restoring health to our bodies, minds, and spirits.

There's a scripture in the Bible that says, "Faith without works is dead" (James 2:26). To me, this means that applying or activating faith implies that one must take action. For instance, you may completely and unreservedly believe that a glass of water will quench your thirst, but until you physically seek out and drink that glass of water, your thirst will not be quenched.

Praying that the water in the glass will help your thirst, understanding in your mind how it can quench your thirst, and then believing in your heart that it will quench your thirst, still won't quench your thirst. It takes that final action step of actually drinking the water.

Where there is no change, there is no life.

While God gives us prayer to use as a tool, we are also designed with brains that can learn and help us make better choices. There are steps we can take that drastically increase our odds of improved health, but we must know what they are, and then take deliberate action steps to implement them into our daily lives. For most of us, it'll take doing things that we're not used to and are probably a little bit out of our comfort zone.

DON'T GET STUCK

Many people simply get into a "rut" where they do the same routines over and over again, pray that things would change, and expect different results. As you've probably heard before, this is the very definition of insanity. I had an old country patient tell me once that "A rut is just a grave with the ends kicked out." It's funny, but it's a pretty true statement that applies to so many areas of our lives. We have to make changes in order to grow.

Where there is no change, there is no life. It's crazy to expect that anything in your life regarding health will change significantly if you don't take some significant steps to actually do something different. It's just so true that you get out of life what you put into it.

That being said, some people do just the opposite. They're on a constantly changing roller-coaster ride of a life without stability, consistency, or balance.

They make wise choices for a few weeks and then totally slip back into a lifestyle that's self-destructive. Regardless of which way they choose, either of these people may "blink and wake up" at age 62 in a hospital room, about to undergo some major, high-risk, life-altering surgery for a critical, life-threatening disease. What happened? They did what all of us do…they got "too busy."

They never took the time to stop, assess where they were in life, and try to identify problematic areas that needed to change. Many times, if they don't change these "problem" areas, it'll end up greatly impacting their lives, and usually in ways that they and their families aren't going to like. In order to achieve the kind of health in life that we all want, we have to STOP at some point and change the path we're on.

THE TWO GROUPS

When my dad and I sit together after a long day's work and chat about our patients, the conversation often drifts to a common theme. When we think about the patients we have who are over the age of 70, we can't help but notice a pattern. There seems to be two really distinct groups of patients. The first group consists of the patients who are fit, routinely get spinal adjustments, are rarely in pain, exercise often, eat well, get plenty of rest, focus on reducing stress, usually take very little medication, travel a great deal, are quite active, enjoy life, have great attitudes, and are typically a whole lot of fun to be around.

As you might imagine, the other group is pretty much the exact opposite. This group of folks tends to be overweight, rarely get adjusted, are frequently in a great deal of pain, hardly ever exercise, eat horribly, have trouble sleeping, are totally stressed out, take a long list of medications, hardly ever get out of the house, have trouble getting around, don't seem to be enjoying life, have horrible or negative attitudes, and are frankly not much fun to be around.

I don't think that this is just coincidental. When you look at how these two groups of people live their lives, it seems pretty obvious why each group gets the health outcome they're experiencing. When you see a pattern over and over again, you can't help but recognize the differences and realize what's going on. As they say, results don't lie!

There was another key difference that really stuck out to me as I pondered these two groups of people. Neither one of these groups are experiencing their particular level of health due to the choices they made last week. They're both receiving either the benefits or consequences of their attitudes and actions toward health later in life as a result of many years of living out their "plan" or lack thereof.

It's no different than a bank account. If we wisely put money in the bank on a weekly basis over 70 years, then at the end, we're really going to like our statement balance! If we don't put anything in until the 69th year, we're going to be severely disappointed with the results. Likewise, going to the gym five days a week is going to create a different outcome than going once a year or even once a month. In order to get the greatest degree of change and to prevent many of the issues that people face as they age, the changes must begin as soon as possible. Seeds planted now reap a harvest somewhere down the road, *not* the next day. Then, those changes must become consistent daily habits.

I watched my mom and dad make great choices in all areas of their health, each of the years I've known them. He's now over the age of 80, still working with patients five days a week, and he clearly fits into that first group we discussed. That's no accident. Less than half of men in America actually reach the age of 80. Can you believe that? That means that the majority of men in America never make it to their 80th birthday![8] My mom is nearly 80 and still exercises with Jazzercise, multiple days per week and is in great shape. She's in that first group, too.

They're reaping the benefits of wise choices or "planting good seeds" early on and along the way. They're still enjoying an amazing quality, as well as quantity, of life. They take no medication and wake up each day with energy, feeling good and are ready to go! Their example makes it clear to me which group I'd like to be in when I'm in my 80's. How about you?

Let me give you a simple, guiding principle for what this book is all about. I believe that God had and still has an Original Design for all people and all things in this universe. Additionally, the further away from the Original Design that we get, the greater our individual and shared problems will become.

Most people feel like health is a seemingly unattainable goal and a difficult puzzle to figure out. It doesn't have to be that way if we have some basic understanding. I believe that there are four basic pieces to this "puzzle" of health. These pieces constitute what I'll refer to from this point on as the four pillars of the foundation of health.

THE FOUR PILLARS

The four pillars of the foundation of health are the major factors that affect health and that can and will be, in this book, broken down into many other parts. These pillars are, however, separate, unique, and critically important, individually. They are mental, physical, chemical, and spiritual.

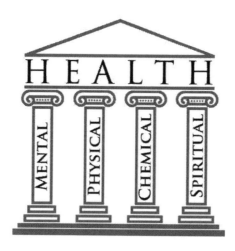

The mental pillar encompasses all the areas of the mind that are intangible and can't be quantified, counted, measured, or documented. This pillar could be subdivided into emotional health, psychological challenges, thoughts, stress, attitudes, good and bad memories, dreams, unforgiveness, beliefs, hopes, etc.

The physical pillar could be subdivided into areas that are tangible and measurable, like spinal and skeletal alignment, blood levels, organ function, exercise, muscle strength, bone density, flexibility, and posture, etc.

The chemical pillar covers everything that involves a substance that enters your body or that your body produces. It could also be subdivided into measurable parts like food, water, air quality, harsh chemical exposure, supplements, drug use, radiation, effects of sleep, hormones, and brain chemicals, etc.

There's not *one* pillar of the foundation of health that's more important than the other.

The spiritual pillar is also intangible and immeasurable. This would be everything that has to do with your faith, your core beliefs, your internal navigator, your spirit, your soul, your place in the universe, your understanding of and relationship with God, prayer, love and how that affects your other three pillars.

While each of the pillars are unique and indispensable, it's extremely interesting to me how many of the factors that influence our health can fit into more than one of the four pillars of health. Take, for instance, exercise. It affects the physical pillar by creating strong muscles, ligaments, and tendons that support your skeletal system. However, exercise also affects the chemical pillar by releasing endorphins that ease pain and make you sweat, which helps cleanse your body of toxins. Exercise affects the mental pillar by helping diminish stress and by creating chemicals in the brain that give you a sense of well-being. The spiritual pillar can also be strengthened by exercise when you realize how amazing the design and function of your body is and that it's a gift from God.

EQUAL PARTS

There's a concept that's not being discussed in many health books these days, and in my estimation it's absolutely critical to understand: There's not *one* pillar of the foundation of health that's more important than the other. So many people are "putting all of their eggs in one basket" by focusing all of their energy and efforts on components of just one or two of the pillars, while virtually ignoring the other two. They may be spending some time on the other two, but they're spending so much *more* time on a few components that they allot very little focus to the others. In doing so, they're completely out of balance and unhealthy.

Let me be clear here: Most people are trying to attain "health" by investing all of their time and effort into the physical and/or chemical pillars of the foundation. Whether they're eating a "healthy" diet or lifting weights or jogging daily or doing yoga or getting massaged and adjusted or taking multiple supplements and/or medications, often they're still just only taking care of one pillar while neglecting the others.

What's interesting is that each pillar of the foundation has a direct effect on each of the other pillars, and each one is vital to our overall health and well-being. In fact, each pillar is *dependent* on the other pillars to create perfect balance. God intended it to be this way; it was and still is the Original Design.

I've seen it time and time again in my practice where patients are doing really well with diet but they never exercise. To make matters worse, they may even sit at a desk all day long and come home only to sit on the couch for the rest of the evening while watching TV. The next day, they get up and do it all over again. Then, they come into my office and tell me about the pain that they're having and relate their frustration about not being healthy. They'll say something like this, "I just don't understand it, Doc. I eat extremely healthily. I don't buy or eat anything that's not at the health food store. Why am I not feeling good? It's not fair!"

While it seems complicated, it's really quite simple. It's much like how the four legs of a stool, when in balance with each other, all hold up the seat. If any leg is shorter than the others, there will be some degree of instability or wobbliness. The shorter the leg, the bigger the wobble and eventually the person may fall. It doesn't matter which leg is shorter; any of them will "rock the boat" if they aren't in balance with the others.

DAWN'S STORY

It reminds me of a patient named Dawn. She was a "perfectly healthy," beautiful, early-20-something-year-old girl who had moved out of state to begin the next chapter in her life. She took good care of her body and did many of the things that we all know are important. Unfortunately, she'd injured her back somehow and explained that she'd been experiencing mid-to lower back pain, abdominal pain, and distension or a swelling on the left side of her "tummy" for over 11 months.

She'd been to multiple specialists over that time and said that she received "many, many misdiagnoses." She was having more and more fatigue associated with it and at one point could barely walk across the room without being exhausted. She eventually had to take a leave of absence from work as she simply could not do her job due to the pain and fatigue.

The doctors told her that her liver was twice its normal size and her spleen had enlarged to *three* times its normal size—it was visibly protruding from her abdomen! Can you imagine what that looked and felt like? She was just a tad concerned. All of the medications and antibiotics that were prescribed for her hadn't changed the situation. Exploratory surgery of the area was being discussed as they just couldn't seem to figure out what was going on.

She flew back home from California, came to our office, and began to receive chiropractic spinal adjustments and supplements that were specific to her condition. Over about two weeks of care, the pain in her back and the swelling in her organs disappeared and that was it—she was all better and ready to get back to her life.

With all of her energy back, Dawn returned to work, feeling great and no longer looked like she was trying to hide a football under her shirt! Although the other areas of her life were in good balance, her physical pillar was failing, and that was causing everything else to crash.

You can imagine how her physical health was affecting her emotional health. Then to be bombarding the body with toxic medications for over 11 months, her chemical pillar was becoming an issue as well. It's easy to see how the pillars of health are all interconnected and how they began to affect one another. Luckily for Dawn, and for many of you, if you get to the root of all of the problems, the balance of health can be restored to its Original Design relatively quickly and easily.

PLANT PILLARS

Another guiding analogy of this book is that of the effect of water, soil, air, and sunlight on plants. These are the four basic needs of a plant to be healthy and thriving. Here's the critical idea to understand: If I were to put a plant in the perfect soil for its species, give it the exact amount of water that it needs, and close it in a dark closet, how healthy will the plant be? Not so healthy, right? In a similar way, if I give it the exact kind of soil and amount of sunlight that it needs, but never water it, how healthy will it be? You got it! Not so healthy. You get the idea. "It ain't rocket science," and yet, it's the very principle that eludes most of us.

You can't say that any one of the requirements of a plant to live healthily is more important than any of the others—they're all essential. Do a poor job of maintaining any of the basic needs of a plant and you may keep the plant alive, but it won't thrive. Depending on the variable that you change, you'll have some different version of the same thing—a sick plant.

This is exactly what we're dealing with in our health today. Some people are doing well with exercise, others are doing well with food, others are doing well emotionally, while others are doing well spiritually. Without creating a balance between all *four* pillars, the foundation of our health is unstable and we experience that as some kind of illness. Our bodies won't be at ease but will be in a state of "dis-ease."

LOOK PAST THE SYMPTOMS

One additional challenge is that, many times in health, what we can see or what we're experiencing is not an accurate representation of what's going on inside of our bodies. It's an extremely false sense of security to think that if we don't feel any symptoms that we're healthy. This, by the way, is why early detection is such an important factor in health. (I would just add that we need early detection of *causes*, not just symptoms!)

Take the following example, which uses one of my favorite sources for analogies—dentistry. Let's say you're bopping along one day, out in the convertible, with the top down, and you and the kids stop for ice cream at the local creamery. You order a scoop of double chocolate fudge ripple, take a big yummy bite, and wham! Like a bolt of lightning, you get a shooting pain in your tooth from a cavity that was already there.

There are several things to discuss here. Do you suppose that when you felt the ice pick-stabbing pain in your face it was the first moment you had that cavity, or had it been building for some time? I think most of us would agree that these things develop over time, and the pain comes at the *end* of the process. To take it one step further, if you were to swish some warm water around in your mouth, it would feel much better, right? Of course it would. The soothing of the warmth overcoming the coldness, and the action of the swishing getting the sugar out of the cavity would bring the irritation to the nerve in the tooth way down.

However, even though you feel fine, is the cavity gone? Of course not. You must get to the underlying cause and remedy *that* in order to regain normal health. Furthermore, regular checkups by your dentist, and discussing your diet and dental hygiene routine, are very important to preventing issues in the first place.

Getting to the very bottom of a problem in any area of health often involves asking the question, "Why?" over and over again until we get to the one true cause of the symptoms. For instance, I had a patient named Janet who came to me with headaches. We discussed all of the issues that she was dealing with, as well as her history of what had happened to her in the past. In her history she related to me that several months prior to the headaches, she'd been getting pain in the neck and shoulders at the end of a long day.

Prior to those pains, she had several years of low back, pelvic, and hip pain. As we dug deeper, she remembered that she had severely sprained her ankle several years before the low back pain started. She recalled limping for months and walking strangely in a boot that stabilized her ankle so it could heal. As we put the pieces of her "puzzle" together, it became clear that after spraining her ankle, walking funny caused her low back, pelvis, and hips to shift into a strange position to compensate for the boot. This began causing the lower half of her body some pain.

As time went on, the neck and upper back began to be strained by the imbalance in her pelvic area. This led to the nerves in her upper neck that go to the head to be irritated and create headaches. Simply taking a pain reliever to help with the pain from the headaches was not going to solve anything long term.

Addressing Janet's current major complaint (headaches) meant getting all the way down to stabilizing the ankle, realigning the pelvis and low back, and working our way up to the middle back and neck, finally strengthening muscles throughout the system to hold everything in place. Getting to the root of the problem is critical!

FIX THE FOUNDATION

Another way to look at it would be with an analogy involving your house. If you had cracks in the ceiling and walls of your home, you could simply patch them up, repaint, and hope for the best—but you know that they'll just come back. If you go down to the concrete foundation, you're likely to find cracks there as well.

In most cases, there's shifting taking place below the foundation, possibly from tree roots, which is the real culprit. To properly deal with this issue, you must remove the tree roots that are affecting the foundation, repair the foundation, repair the walls, repair the ceiling, and then repaint. It also has to be in that specific order, too, or you won't get the results you're looking for. Sadly, we've been trained (usually by people trying to sell us something) to look at the symptoms and then find a treatment for just that one issue, instead of looking at what could be causing it.

We have to take a more comprehensive approach to our health by looking at *all* four pillars of the foundation. We then need to seek out the Original Design for each component of those pillars and attempt to create balance with them. We've got to stop patching things with temporary solutions and begin to look at the foundational issues that are destroying the health of the human race.

**Don't compare your inside
to someone else's outside!**

YOU'RE AN ORIGINAL

One final point that I'd like to present in this Introduction is the other half of Original Design. We discussed quite a bit about the importance of the design of the body, but I want to focus on the original part now.

Listen…you're an original! Don't compare your inside to someone else's outside! People don't show you what's going on inside of them; they only show you what they want you to see. Don't be fooled by their "social media face." Nobody's perfect; we all have issues. Just like there are no two snowflakes that are alike, there are no two humans who are alike…by design. There's only one you! You'll never achieve what you were designed to achieve or be the person you were designed to be while comparing yourself to others. So don't try to be someone else; be you!

You're an original who is capable of doing something incredibly unique that only you can do. Like a highly specialized tool in the kit of a carpenter, you were designed with a specific purpose. Each tool is incredibly valuable and serves the carpenter well when used in the way that it was designed to be used.

Isn't it funny how, in the world, you'll hear the phrase that someone is "such a tool," implying that they're being used? When we understand what we've been designed for, we *want* to be used by God as a tool in His hands. It's the opposite of how it's perceived normally. Tools don't need to understand the details of what's being built; they just need to let the master carpenter use them for their designed purpose. Hammers don't read blueprints…they just pound nails. I'm proud to be a tool. How 'bout you?

There may be others who have similar gifts or talents or looks or mental capacities or physical capabilities or learned skills, but no one, and I mean *no one*, can do it like *you* can. You have to understand this and believe it in your heart of hearts—at your very core!

We all have our role to play in the "body." Some are hands, some are eyes, some are voices, and some are hearts. We will be in constant frustration if we keep trying to be a mouth when we were designed to be an ear. Find your role by seeking God and discovering what you're naturally passionate about. We're all counting on you to do what you were originally designed to do! It's like all the dials and parts of a Swiss watch—they're all important and depend on each other. Everything just works better when all of the parts work together, as originally designed.

We'll talk about some basic needs of all humans as it applies to diet, exercise, sleep, etc., but your specific needs are unique to you. There's no way that one diet can be the perfect diet for all of us, nor can we all have the same job, etc. Think about it. What in nature can you point to that would lead you to believe that we all fit into one box? That's crazy talk! Nature is full of huge variations and slight differences that create uniqueness and beauty. Don't worry about what other people do or have, but focus on who you are and what you've been given. You're an amazing person who is unlike anyone else on the planet! You and I are not accidents.

As I began to understand this concept and formed my ideas for this book, it hit me really hard and I had a few tears. I was designed to write this book and was made to be used as a tool in the hands of God to help certain people achieve the kind of health that they were originally designed to experience. I even changed my license plate to read "ORIGNL" after having this epiphany.

Do I claim to know everything? Of course not. In fact, I always say that the more I learn about health, the more I realize that it's a constant learning process. Do I cover everything there is to know about health in this book? No.

But I have helped thousands of patients in my practice and I want people to know that there's hope their health, peace, and happiness.

Are there other books out there that tell you how to be healthy? Yes, others have written health books—really good ones, in fact. However, this book will resonate with certain people in a way that no other book could.

You too have a purpose that is based on your Original Design that is unique to only you. Seek it and you'll find it!

THE GOOD NEWS AND THE BAD NEWS

In summary, what I hope to accomplish in this book can be summed up in two main points: the bad news and the good news. Here's the bad news first: We need to realize that we're in the middle of a major health crisis on this planet, and we need to understand what we're doing wrong. We're creating most of our own problems at an astounding rate and we've got to stop it. We're well on the way to wiping out our own species.

Here's the good news: If we understand some basic principles of health, balance, and the Original Design, analyze where we're at in our lives (specifically, regarding balance), make a plan of action, and implement it, then we can achieve the level of health we've always dreamed of and always hoped was possible. We can actually reverse much of the damage that we've created to our own health.

A new field of study called epigenetics shows that "our diets and lifestyles can change the expression of our genes, by influencing a network of chemical switches within our cells...."[9] This means that even if you have some genetic predisposition to health problems like diabetes and cardiovascular disease, you don't necessarily have to experience them! Now that's hope!

We can regain our health and get out of the rut we're in! It starts now, and it starts with you and me. The choices we make, the foods we buy, the products we demand in the marketplace, and the life we choose to live will have ripple effects.

These ripple effects will determine things like public policy through influence of politicians, over time what is considered "the norm" as people change their mindsets, and what's on the shelves at the grocery store as companies listen to the products that are being demanded. Ripple effects influence our health, the health of our children and the generations to come.

Never give up believing that your life and the lives of those around you can be better, even when it seems that all of the odds are stacked against you. If you can believe it, you can achieve it!

HOW TO PROCEED

There are two ways to read this book: the old-fashioned way (the best way) where you read from beginning to end, *or*, if you're the impatient type, read the turbo nutshell quick-start synopsis at the end, get started immediately making changes, and then read the rest of the book more slowly, the normal way, as you travel the journey toward health. I encourage you to highlight words or sentences in the book that really jump out at you as you're reading. It's no accident that they're really speaking to you. It's something that you know, on the inside, is important to think about. Now…get reading!

CHAPTER 1

IN THE BEGINNING...

In the beginning... God had an Original Design for everything. According to the Bible, "In the beginning God created the heavens and the earth" (Genesis 1:1). Genesis 1:26 goes on to say: "Then God said, 'Let Us make man in Our image, according to Our likeness; let them have dominion over the fish of the sea, over the birds of the air, and over the cattle, over all the earth and over every creeping thing that creeps on the earth.'"

After God created Adam and Eve, Genesis 1:28 says, "Then God blessed them, and God said to them, 'Be fruitful and multiply; fill the earth and subdue it; have dominion over the fish of the sea, over the birds of the air, and over every living thing that inhabits the earth.'" And when renewing His covenant with Noah some time later, God said, "*Everything* that lives and moves about will be food for you. Just as I gave you the green plants, I now give you everything" (Genesis 9:3 NIV).

"In the beginning" of this book I want us all to agree on a very crucial and core principle. Without this principle as a foundation, it will be difficult for any of the rest of this book to truly make sense. The principle is this: There is a God who had, and who still has, a plan for everyone and everything in the universe.

God's not dumb. He is supreme intelligence. Everything in our world works together in amazing ways; it's hard to deny that it was designed to work that way. The body that He designed isn't dumb, either. It's extremely intelligent and is designed to work in a beautifully harmonious way, such that we have abundant life and unbelievable capabilities to thrive, to create, to help, and to heal.

Everything in the universe has a purpose and fits together beautifully in a symphony of movement and harmony when allowed to work in the way that it was originally designed. Humans, though, have changed so many things from the way they began that we have severely altered the way things are designed to work, and the results have had devastating consequences.

The good news is that nearly everything we've altered or damaged to problematic extents can be restored back to what it was originally designed to be. Built into most of all designed things is the capacity for restoration. That's also part of the Original Design…it all is.

We're the happiest, healthiest, and feel the most fulfilled when we're doing what we were designed to do.

DESIGN JUST MAKES SENSE

Considering that about 90% of us on planet earth believe in God, it's safe to say that I've only lost about 10% of you so far. Just wait! Stick with me for a minute, my atheist friends. I think even the 10% will find a ton of wisdom here, as well as current and historical information from studies, research, and life experience to back up what I'm about to get into.

If, as an atheist or agnostic person, you can't believe in an Original Designer, you can still recognize the value and beauty of design. Nearly everything that you see in this world or use in your life has a specific purpose, and when used in the correct way it's the most effective and valuable. Design just makes sense. For instance, you might be able to slowly hammer in a nail with a screwdriver, but that screwdriver was simply not designed to put in nails! When you use it as a hammer, it's weak and ineffective. However, when you use it for its intended purpose, or what it was designed for, it works extremely well. That's all part of the Original Design for that tool. Likewise, we're the happiest, healthiest, and feel the most fulfilled when we're doing what *we* were designed to do.

So many things in this life work just like that. They work so much better when they're used in the way that they were intended to be used. It's simply looking at things in our lives and evaluating them by the measuring stick of Original Design that helps to keep us all on track. So even if you choose not to believe that there is an Original Designer, you can still benefit from the idea of Original Design because it applies to nearly everything in your life. The truth is, the further we get away from the Original Design for anything, the bigger the mess we get ourselves in to.

For example, let's talk about the drift away from the Original Design of food. This is an easy one that we all see every day, and most of us already know it. Take fruit, not genetically modified in any way, which is grown organically, in its intended environment, under ideal growing conditions of light, water, air, and soil; and it ripens "on the vine," so to speak. Then, let's say, you eat it at the peak of maturity and freshness. It'll be so good, so tasty, so sweet, so fragrant, and so nutritious. It'll be amazing to enjoy *and* incredibly healthy for your body!

Now let's deviate it from the Original Design just a little. Pick a variable—any variable. Stray from the optimal conditions and the fruit's overall taste, health value, etc., will suffer. What if you grow it in an area that it barely has time to mature, or doesn't get enough water, or sunlight? Not as good, right? What if you spray it with pesticides, pick it early, store it for months, and gas it to artificially "ripen" it? Mmm, sounds yummy. Can I have some please? No way!

What if, after harvesting, you chop it up, boil it, add preservatives, mix it with fillers, artificial colors, and other chemicals, and mold it into "fruit snacks" in all sorts of cool shapes and package it in the cheapest chemical-laden plastic known to man, box it, and put it on a shelf for a year or so, and then eat it? Are you kidding me? What kind of a warped nightmare is that? Unfortunately, many Americans and people all around the world in "modernized" cities are, in fact, kidding themselves if they think they can severely alter things in the world around them without creating negative consequences.

Make no mistake about it: The further we alter a food, or *anything*, from its Original Design, the more we suffer. Even if the effects of the alterations take time to accumulate before being seen, it's still happening.

SIDE EFFECTS

Research seems to always show the effect of something that took so long to detect, that by the time we figure it out it's either too late or severe damage has already been done. Don't you love it when the FDA takes a drug off the market; many years later, only *after* hundreds of people have been severely injured or died?

If you look back, though, you'll always see how that drug created a clear shift away from the originally designed function of the body. It may temporarily create a "desirable" effect, but in the end that alteration ends up creating the "side effect" problem. It's often trying to force the body to do something that it just wasn't designed to do. It's a short-sighted "patch" that has a long list of side effects because it messes with the designed function of the system as a whole. One thing seems to get better but everything else gets thrown off.

This reminds me of a patient named Sally, who had slightly elevated cholesterol of around 220. Her doctor was very persistent in getting her to take a common cholesterol-lowering medication known as a statin drug. It blocks the production of cholesterol in the liver, which theoretically lowers your cholesterol number on a blood test. Your liver produces cholesterol normally because it's an important precursor or foundational ingredient to making hormones that you *need* and is a critical part of every cell membrane on earth. The problem, of course, is that when you "poison" the body with a drug and cause it to *dys*function or not function the way it was originally designed, then other issues arise.

WebMD says that side effects of statin drugs can include intestinal problems, liver damage, muscle inflammation and pain, memory loss, mental confusion, high blood sugar, and type 2 diabetes. I've seen patients in my practice with every single one of those side effects over the years.

So, as time went by, Sally indeed lowered her cholesterol "number" a few points but began to have other issues and pains. When she went back to the doctor to see what was going on, they did more blood work and found that her liver enzyme numbers were sky high and that she was having early liver failure. Their recommendation was to have her get off of the statin drug immediately. Sounds like a good idea to me. Duh.

Within a month or so, her blood work was normal and she was feeling much better. What was their suggestion at that point? You guessed it— go back on the statin drug to keep the cholesterol down. Hmmm. No thanks! I'm not even convinced that her mildly "elevated" numbers were an issue as the "normal" value was considered to be below 250 until 2004 when the American Heart Association lowered its recommended level to below 200.

The point of this story is that when we alter anything from its Original Design, in this case we're talking about the function of the liver, there will always be an effect that we may not like. When things function the way they were designed to, however, we will always get the ideal result. In Sally's case, some dietary changes, supplements, and exercise helped her body heal and function normally, which caused her cholesterol numbers to reduce *on their own*. Heal the system and watch everything fall into place.

Let me take time right now to make something very clear, though: I'm not a basher of the medical community and medical doctors—quite the opposite, in fact. I work hand in hand with great medical doctors every day in my office toward a common goal of helping people.

Sally's doctor wasn't doing anything wrong, and in actuality was doing exactly what he was required to do as a licensed medical physician. There's something that all of us doctors are bound to, which is called the "standard of care." If her MD had not recommended that Sally go on the statin drug, and she would've had some sort of cardiovascular problem like a heart attack or stroke, he could've been sued for improperly informing and not treating her condition based on current standards. In a way, there's little choice for a doctor but to suggest what the current, accepted treatment is for any given condition. Side effects are simply a well-known problem with all medicines, as we have all seen on the TV commercials that spend more time listing *them* than they do talking about the benefits of the drug.

Medical doctors and the medical profession in the United States of America are second to none, and we are fortunate to have them. Seriously, would you rather get really sick in a third-world jungle or in the US? I always tell patients, "If I get run over by a truck, I don't want a chiropractic adjustment and some supplements! I want the best surgeons in America, and some really heavy drugs!" What I simply want us to refocus on is to strive to restore our bodies to their Original Design so they can function at their maximum capacity, on their own, without the need for drugs that could create harm.

GOOD PROGRESS IS GOOD

Now I want to stop those of you whose minds are going down the path of, "I suppose he thinks progress is wrong, computers are a bad idea, cars and planes just pollute the air, credit cards are evil, we should avoid all medications, JFK's assassins were never caught, and Elvis is still alive." To use an old Texas saying, "Hold yer horsies there, buckaroo!"

Progress *is* an Original Design, and I'm no conspiracy theorist. I'm more of a realist. You've heard it said that the only thing that remains constant is that everything changes. I believe there was always the design and intention for change and of being presented with a challenge and finding a solution. This is a built-in, genetic piece of our design that's part of what makes us human.

As a species, we're always trying to find solutions to life's challenges and mysteries, to improve things and make life better or easier. However, I think my wife would sometimes like me to stop finding solutions and start listening. "You don't always need to fix it! I just need you to listen, my love!" she'll say. I can hear her now.

Clearly, many things are not as they were "in the beginning," and it's a good thing that some of them changed. Indoor plumbing and sewage systems with treatment plants and appropriate disposal are good things. They've helped stop severe plagues when germ transmission was at an all-time high in medieval days when sewage was simply dumped in the streets. Gross, dude!

Some changes have not been good, though. When we began engineering "foods" and altering them severely from their originally designed state and infusing them with chemicals that extend shelf life and made them taste "better," we made a large, even fatal, error. Still more things could, will, and should change, but within certain guidelines.

Technology and advancement are wonderful and amazing things, and for the most part can be really good for humanity. It just shouldn't be at the expense of human health or the destruction of the planet. There's an appropriate time, way, and place for growth and change. If we don't follow a time-tested and, in my opinion, God-authored plan, we'll be trying to do things based on our own limited knowledge and experience, not the Original Design. Are we so cavalier to believe that we could or even should try to fix what isn't broken?

It reminds me of a scene in one of my favorite movies, *Contact*, where some higher power has sent a message through space that has the blueprints for a time-travel machine encoded in it. It's a massive, extremely complex, multibillion-dollar machine with millions of moving parts. As the scientists begin to assemble this machine, they determine that the pod that carries the time traveler in it "isn't good enough." And so decide they need to install a restraint system and a flight chair and other devices to make it "safe."

Think about that. Some infinitely more intelligent being has sent them the exact plans for a time machine that is designed perfectly for its intended purpose, but the scientists decide that *they* know better. (I'm laughing right now.) Are you serious?! Well, they start the huge machine, and it begins to spin and create all of this bright light and energy, and the "astronaut," played by Jodie Foster, says, "I'm picking up a moderate vibration here," to which the lead scientist reassuringly says, "The vibration is normal." As if he knows! He didn't design it!

The vibration gets worse and she says, "Vibration is getting a little stronger now." The lead scientist turns to one of his assistants, who tells him, "We're detecting some structural instability, but we're within limits…barely." Again, how would he know? So they launch the pod into the time machine. Foster's character experiences a falling sensation and appears to drop into a time/space tunnel or wormhole. As she goes along, the shaking of her chair and equipment intensifies until it's unbearable. She frees herself from the harness and is immediately peacefully floating inside the pod with *zero* vibration.

The chair and equipment eventually break apart and fall away. Now it's totally calm inside the pod, the way it was *designed* to be, and she's totally fine. All they had to do was trust the original design of the blueprints freely given to them by this vastly more intelligent being.

Sound familiar? When we try to "improve" on something that was already designed perfectly by the Original Designer because we think we know better, we often create our own problems, and may go so far as to even get mad at Him. The writer of Proverbs said, "A person's own folly leads to their ruin, yet their heart rages against God" (Proverbs 19:3 NIV). All that's actually required of us is to trust the Original Design and the One who freely gave it to us in the first place.

For instance, do any of us honestly believe that we're going to engineer a food that's healthier than what God put on the planet for us to eat? Does anyone really think that they understand how to navigate through life better than the One who designed life in the first place? When you think about it, it's ridiculous and just plain silly.

Motives for alteration of anything from its Original Design need to be severely scrutinized. Most of the time, we simply don't *need* to "reinvent the wheel." God designed a way for this world and everything in it to work. Trust in that. We can try to fit the proverbial square peg in the round hole, but wouldn't it just make more sense to put the square peg in the square hole? It's easier, reduces stress, creates joy because of how smoothly it works, and has no collateral damage.

Trusting in the Original Design is so freeing! You don't have to try to navigate through and decipher all of the intricate details of life. Trust in what God designed and what He said and it will work out great! For example, if you trust that God knows what job is best for you, then you simply look, apply, and wait. You don't have to stress out about it because you know that God will cause the job to work out that was designed for you. Becoming and staying healthy can also be stressful and confusing unless you do one thing: look to what God made. Simple.

It's hard to deny the truths that are so evident all around us. Veering from the Original Design can create (and has already created) myriad issues for the human race and the planet as a whole. Deviating from the Original Design, in fact, can have and has had everywhere from small to massive consequences.

RESTORATION

I've often thought that had I been responsible for creating the human body, I would've made it far less forgiving. To my brain, if you treat your body unhealthily by smoking four packs of cigarettes a day, drinking a bottle of whiskey, and eating donuts all day long, then you should probably self-destruct and explode somewhere around 21 years of age.

The good news for all of us is that I didn't create the human body. God did. The body was designed to be much more durable and capable of adapting to less-than-ideal circumstances, and it's amazingly capable of actually healing itself. What have humans created that can live, breathe, and heal itself? We're good, but we aren't nearly as good as God.

Most all things can change, and much of what we've damaged is not ruined but is simply not in the state that it was designed to be. Over time, it can be turned in the direction of or even restored back to its Original Design. All of our cells, our organs, our bodies, our relationships, our emotional "hearts," and many things on our planet even, have been designed to be remarkably resilient and have the ability to slowly (and occasionally quickly) be restored. It's amazing!

That always blows me away! It's such great news. It's like waking up from a nightmare and realizing that, in reality, everything is not the disaster that you were anticipating and that it's all going to be okay. Whew! What a relief!

Pretty much all of you gardeners can attest to the transformation of a neglected, bone-dry plant that appeared to be totally dead. Most people will just throw them away, but occasionally you take a liking to a particular plant and decide to revive it. So you cut the plant back to its base, repot it in good soil, water it regularly, and give it the kind of sunlight and fresh air that it needs. It doesn't come back overnight, but after a period of time (a different amount for different plants), it slowly begins to show signs of life.

**Take what's been damaged in any area of your life,
get refocused on doing what was originally
designed to be done, and watch the "magic"
of restoration take place!**

First, there may be only a little green note to the coloring of the plant, and then with time, the roots heal, grow, and then you get a tiny shoot of growth. With more time, a leaf forms, then two, and then a hundred! Suddenly it's coming back to life—a far cry from where it was, all sad, pitiful looking, and worthless. Eventually, it begins to look like it did before it was neglected, and perhaps it may even look better—yes *better*—than it did when you first got it. And then, the miracle of miracles...the plant begins to flower and even bear fruit! What once was considered trash and was about to be discarded, is now vibrantly healthy, beautiful, life-giving, and valuable.

This story could practically be about anything in your life that needs work. This is such an exciting aspect of how Original Design works. Take what's been damaged in any area of your life, get refocused on doing what was originally designed to be done, and watch the "magic" of restoration take place! It's so beautiful. You may be experiencing some significant health challenges and feeling sad, pitiful and worthless, yourself. But if you're rooted in the Original Design, you can bounce back.

After reading that analogy of the plant, some of you may be thinking about your physical health issues. Some of you may be thinking about a relationship in trouble; while others of you may be thinking about previous damage to your spiritual health. And a few of you are thinking, "You know, I really need to go water my actual plants in the backyard right now." ☺

However it affected you, the core idea is still the same. There are steps you can take to change a situation involving nearly any area of your health. A real transformation can take place that restores your health completely back to or really close to its Original Design.

You can't rewrite the beginning of your story, but you can change the ending.

Listen, I understand. There's a lot of confusion out there. When I give talks or classes on any aspect of health, there are always people at the end who come up to me with tons of questions. Everyone has things they know they want to change, but they don't know how. That's why I wrote this book. I want to give people any knowledge or wisdom I might have that can help guide them toward a healthier future. It can be done! I've seen it over and over again!

I want you to say this to yourself right now: "I can change. This isn't who I was designed to be and it's not how I was designed to live. I'm done accepting mediocrity. I was made for more than this! I must and I will regain my Original Design! Change starts now. I will be healthy!" You can't rewrite the beginning of your story, but you can change the ending.

CHAPTER 2

BALANCE

When we consider our lives, we all have a slightly different idea of what constitutes success or happiness, but we all tend to agree that we feel better overall when things are in "balance." Balance is truly one of the keys that we all strive for, whether or not we know it. When each aspect of your life is experiencing some level of success, you'll find that all four pillars of health are in balance.

Have you ever put the middle of a long stick on your outstretched finger and tried to get it to balance without tipping one way or the other? The exact balance point is different for each stick, but *every* stick has a point of balance. Our health is similar—the point of balance may be different than someone else's, but we can all find balance in our lives.

If you're well adjusted, exercising, eating well, drinking plenty of water, getting good rest, spending time with family, enjoying work, taking time to play, and spiritually fulfilled, you'll experience good health. The exact details of each of those components of health are unique to you. However, the more of these areas that are out of sync with what you want for your life (or more importantly, what you *need* in your life), then you'll feel anxiety, fear, anger, depression, and any of the other negative emotions that come as a result. It's easy to say, "Get everything in balance, and you'll be happy!" But as we all know, "it ain't that easy!"

When each aspect of your life is experiencing some level of success, you'll find that all four pillars of health are in balance.

LOOKS CAN BE DECEIVING

Let me tell you a story about a patient of mine named Mike. To look at him on the outside, you'd think he was extremely healthy and "balanced." Mike was a great guy, 44 years old, great sense of humor, athletic and "fit" looking. He worked out at the gym at least five days per week and was what you might call "ripped." With his big biceps, chiseled chest, and "six pack" abs, he could've done the cover of a men's fitness magazine.

The problem was that Mike absolutely hated his job and would frequently come in to the office steaming, even "shaking mad," about some issue at work, his boss, or a coworker. He was also stressed at home as he and his wife were having significant marital problems, which caused him to miss sleep. To add fuel to the fire, he ate whatever junk food he wanted, whenever he wanted. He often came to the office eating fast food and a big soda after his workout and would hurriedly stuff it in his mouth right before his adjustment.

Mike and I would have discussions in the office about his diet and he would say, "Doc, come on, man, look at me. Do I look like I need to be on a diet?" His perception was that a "diet" was for "fat" people and it gave him visions of small-portion frozen dinners and "low fat" prepackaged foods, boring salads, powdered shakes, or steamed veggies.

Of course he looked great on the *outside*, but health goes deeper than appearance. I could never get him to accept that there was a connection between what we eat and how we function, how we feel, and ultimately, our overall health. Time and time again we'd casually discuss his high-stress level at work and home, his sleep deficit, and his junky diet. Like most of us, it was much the same week to week.

That was until one day when he missed his appointment. I found out later that day, that while at the gym with his 18 year-old son, just prior to their workout, he had a major heart attack and passed away right there. It was discovered that he had severe blockage of several major arteries due to cardiovascular disease. Mike totally bought into the idea that working out and getting the occasional spinal adjustment would keep him feeling good and would "save" him from any health issues that might show up in the course of his life. He did, of course, enjoy some improved health with exercise and chiropractic care, but obviously he still had some major areas of his overall health that were severely neglected.

HEALTH IS BALANCE

We must consider health as the balance of *all* of the pillars of the foundation of health, and not simply focus on only one or two areas really diligently. As you've heard, "Life is a journey, not a destination." We have to do some things to learn how to enjoy each minute we've been given. We can't look to the future so much that we overlook what's in front of us or live in the past so much that we miss what's ahead.

We need to stay "in the moment," keep our focus on what's important, and let go of what's not. Look, none of us can ever achieve a state of perfection. To have that expectation would be self-defeating, will set you up for failure, and it could create a state of depression.

In life, much of the pain we feel is from unmet expectations. This certainly doesn't mean to set your expectations low, but to have expectations that allow for a certain degree of flexibility, especially with certain situations or seasons of your life. You can achieve a state of balance where you're handling life's seasonal challenges and triumphs with peace and stability.

SEASONS IN LIFE

"What are seasons?" you might ask. I'm not talking about spring, summer, fall, and winter, of course. The seasons I'm talking about are time periods in your life that change based on what's going on around you. You have a season as a child, a single adult, a married couple without children, then with children, then without children (in the house) again, and sometimes, unfortunately, without your spouse and single again.

You then experience seasons within those seasons, like during times of a heavy workload, family stress, serving at your church, being involved in various organizations, times of bad health, and the list goes on. Each season should have expectations of its own, which should not be confused with other seasons.

For example, let's say that you were on a good stretch and finally exercising like you want to, and then you get sick. As long as you're in this "mini-season" of being sick, you'd get out of balance, so to speak, by not exercising during that period. Due to the circumstances of that season, you'd purposefully change the balance and put more focus on rest, and that's okay. In fact, it's critical to healing in *that* season of life.

You've heard the terms "roll with the punches" or "go with the flow." During certain seasons you need to do just that; plan for the best case scenario, but if it doesn't work out, have the ability to let it go and not get caught up in what didn't go right. I'd even suggest that being upset about that unmet expectation can easily cause you to lose focus for the next thing to come.

If a professional basketball player misses a shot and gets really down on himself, he's in the wrong mental state for the next shot. He has to be able to learn from the mistake if possible, let it go, and be mentally ready for the next opportunity. Many a game in sports has been won by the team or player who stayed mentally focused, even when it seemed like they were going to lose.

We too need to have a "reset button" that mentally puts the past behind us and gives us a fresh start for the next season. Yes, we learn from the challenges that we endure, but we can't focus on the challenge and stay in the pain associated with it. We have to let it go, or we'll never be able to move forward.

PEOPLE ARE LIKE PLANTS

One of my favorite analogies of balance involving plants, previously discussed in the Introduction, is one that even little kids understand and learn in grade school at an early age. In second grade, we did "experiments" on bean seeds, and then later, the seedlings that came from them. First, our entire class got a little cup and some potting soil and a few beans to plant in the soil. We watered our little beans and put them on a big tray by the window with the brightest, warmest sunshine.

Over time, the beans began to sprout and we all had these happy, healthy little plants that looked nearly identical. At this point, however, we began to change up the variables. Some would put the seedling in a sandy soil, some in a more clay-like soil, and some in the same rich soil that they sprouted in. Then each of the three soil groups were divided into three other groups that watered either too little, too much, or an ideal amount. After several weeks, some had died, many were sickly, but some were quite healthy. Last, the healthy ones were then subjected to one hour, four hours, or a full day of sunlight.

In the end, there were a few clear winners. The ones with the ideal balance of soil, water, and sunlight were huge, green, and strong plants. One of the plants was even flowering and ready to make more beans. The balance of all of the factors was critical! Are you following me?

The analogy to our lives is obvious. When all of the variables that affect our health are in proper balance, we thrive and become "fruitful" ourselves.

What I've since discovered, now that I'm "all growed up," is that my grade-school bean experiment would've been different with a different seed. All seeds and the plants they become require different conditions to be healthy. Each plant has unique needs to mature correctly, be healthy, blossom, and bear fruit.

Like plants, all of us have basic needs, but the details vary slightly from person to person. Each of us has a unique and Original Design, like every seed or plant. All plants need some kind of foundation, like soil, water, air, and sunlight. However, the exact mixture of nutrients and pH of the soil varies. The amount, pH, and nutrient value of the water varies. The amount of air and the exact mixture of altitude and carbon dioxide all vary. The amount, timing, and intensity of sunlight will also vary. All of these factors have specific requirements to produce a healthy specimen of that particular plant.

We, as humans, all need healthy food, clean water, ample rest, normal nerve function, emotional health, structural stability, spiritual strength, muscle strength, oxygen, and a long list of things that are required to keep us alive. It is, however, the precise quantity and quality of these factors that determines our health, happiness, and the quality of our lives.

INTERDEPENDENT PILLARS

Interestingly, some of the needs of humans fit into multiple categories. For instance, let's take exercise. Exercise obviously fits into the physical pillar because, when we do it, we build strength in our muscles, tendons, and ligaments, and it causes our bones to become denser. Overall, our structure or frame becomes stronger.

Exercise also fits into the chemical category because, when we exercise, our bodies produce endorphins that act as painkillers, adrenaline that gives us energy, serotonin that helps us sleep, and lactic acid that's a result of the breakdown of the muscles. Additionally, exercise fits nicely into the mental pillar because research shows that people who exercise report less stress, greater emotional stability, less anxiety and depression, and better cognitive or thinking abilities.

Another example of how the balance of health is affected by the interdependence between pillars is with nutrition. There are times when nutrition is so badly out of balance that we have an inability to handle things, mentally or emotionally, because of some nutrient deficiency. This commonly happens when fat soluble vitamins, hormones, minerals, and many other nutrients are out of balance due to poor diet.

Very few people realize this, but vitamin D is actually a steroid hormone. That's right. It's a hormone! It can greatly affect your emotions (among many other things). Studies done on rats that have been deprived of certain nutrients show how easily confused, agitated, and panicky they can become when given a maze or some other problem to solve.

I have a good friend who has a chemical pillar imbalance called hypoglycemia. When he hasn't eaten anything in a while, and his blood sugar drops too low, he can get shaky, agitated, and act very strangely. One day when we met at a restaurant and he'd barely eaten anything all day, he became frustrated with our server for not bringing out our complimentary bread fast enough. He got on her about it just a little bit too hard and kind of yelled at her to bring the bread! She did so quite quickly, and as it hit the table he hastily grabbed a piece and then proceeded to take a voracious bite…only he missed the bread and bit his finger. Now that's a chemical imbalance! But I'll bet our server just thought he had a mental imbalance!

**All of the factors that affect health
intertwine to create a harmonious balance
and support for each other.**

SOLUTIONS TO IMBALANCES

One challenging thing about health care is that, many times, in seeking a solution, people have to do a lot of trial and error with trying different doctors, therapists, and techniques until they find the unique combination of treatments that works for them with their specific body type and set of circumstances. I can attest personally, and by the reports of thousands of patients, that it's usually some combination of techniques and treatments that will be necessary to conquer the difficult issues and restore balance back to one's health. It makes sense when you think about it.

How likely is it that all of our health issues are going to be solved by *one* health-care professional or diet or exercise class? More than likely, the greatest degree of balance will be found in our health as we address *all* of the areas that we'll discuss in this book.

All of the factors that affect health intertwine to create a harmonious balance and support for each other. They're interdependent pieces of an intricate puzzle that we call health. You can't claim that one piece of it is more important than another anymore than you can say the heart is more important than the brain, the liver, or the stomach. All of the pieces are different, but the "picture of health" is incomplete without all of the pieces.

Let's say you have a plant that's sickly and barely hanging on to life because you're only giving it just enough sunlight or water to make it another day. You'll never have that plant be the vibrant, healthy specimen it was originally designed to be unless you learn all of the specific requirements *it* needs to thrive, and then actually provide them to the plant on a daily basis.

As humans, we must first look at the Original Design and learn everything that we, as *unique* individuals, need to be healthy. Next, we must create a prioritized list of areas that we need to focus on improving. Then, once we take action steps to implement our list or plan, balance, optimal health and a sense of well-being will become ours. These are the three easy steps that we'll discuss more at the end of the book.

PILLAR I

MENTAL

CHAPTER 3

PERCEPTION AND ATTITUDE

COMMUNICATION

When two people are retelling a story, they may have two completely different versions and yet both of them are telling the "truth." Their versions of the story are based on what they remember or their perception of what happened. They're telling it just like it is, in *their* minds, and could pass lie detector tests concerning the details of their perception of the story. Perception is at the core of what we experience as reality.

Reality for each person is based on that perception, and that, in turn, determines his or her attitude. How things are communicated to us, like voice inflection, body language, word choice, the emotional state we're in at the time, experiences from the past, and what we want to hear, are just a few of the things that greatly shade our perception. In fact, one researcher found that 55% of communication between people is done by nonverbal cues, like body language, eye contact, facial expression, etc., 38% is voice tone, and only 7% of the communication is the actual words being said.[1] Our perception of what is said is absolutely directed by these other factors.

This is why e-mails, texts and social media posts can create some serious misperceptions that can cause confusion and anger.

Try actually talking to someone in person every now and then. It's quite refreshing. Hey, even video conferencing allows you to actually see the person and hear their voice. It's extremely convenient and as close to reality as technology can provide. In the end, the only way that you can clear up misperception is by better communication. At the center of all failed businesses, relationships, or anything involving multiple people, is poor communication. Nothing will change without people communicating clearly, with love, honesty, and patience. I've personally done a good job at damaging relationships in the past by not communicating the way I just described. Fail.

ROOTS OF PERCEPTION

Perception is definitely based on the experiences that have happened to you over time and how you were raised. For instance, you might've grown up in a healthy family, where junk food was never allowed and explained to you as being really "bad." So now when you see someone give a bag of candy to their kid, you might judge that person and think how irresponsible of a parent they are and perceive that parent to be harming or even abusing their child.

On the other hand, what if you were raised in a family where bags of candy were given as a prize to celebrate something that had been accomplished? You might view that same situation and think what a great parent that person is for rewarding their children. One single event can evoke extremely different thoughts and emotions in different people.

Let's look at how perception affects your everyday life when viewed through the eyes of people at different ends of the spectrum. If you perceive that everyone in the world is out to get you, then you're likely to live a life that's guarded, pessimistic, skeptical, cynical, and negative. This kind of person is often called "street smart" or even "jaded."

What if you're at the other extreme of perception? This is where you're optimistic and perceive everyone to be loving, understanding, moral, and trustworthy. Unfortunately, you may be easily duped, abused, and otherwise taken advantage of in some way. These people are often considered to be naïve. Now, of course, we all have to have *some* measuring stick by which to analyze or judge the world around us. Neither is the right way, but it's simply a by-product of genetics, experiences, and upbringing.

Naturally, there's a happy medium between the two extremes I just described. The Bible says that we are to be "as shrewd as snakes and as innocent as doves" (Matthew 10:16 NIV). I would say that we should strike a balance between guarding our hearts and being cautious while believing the best about people and giving them the benefit of the doubt. My dad says it something like this: "In business, it's always best to do arm's-length transactions that give you a little bit of room to maneuver." This gives you room in case you should need to get out of it, but you're close enough to be kind and genuine.

It's funny. It reminds me of a dance we held at a Christian youth camp. Teenagers dancing too closely to each other can give a panic attack to parents and counselors trying to keep everyone in line. They'd put about two feet between us, where your hands could just reach the shoulders of your dance partner, but not close enough to have bodies touching. One counselor said we needed to "leave room between us for the Holy Spirit."

However you slice it, you have to leave some room in your mind before you make a permanent decision about anyone or anything that's solely based on your perception instead of "all the facts." Others have said it like this, "Hope for the best but prepare for the worst." In the end, you may need someone to be slow to judge you, so try to do the same for them.

ATTITUDE

Let me tell you one of my favorite stories about Joker and Sam. Joker was the family dog, a collie-sheepdog mix that I got when I turned one.

We formed a very strong bond and she followed me everywhere. Sam was the black-and-white family cat that we inherited from my eldest sister after college. He, like all cats, was independent, but he was usually very loving.

This story about Joker and Sam played out dozens of times over the years because of where we live. In central Texas, thunderstorms, especially in spring, are common and can be incredibly violent. The storms often have high winds, driving rain, and, of course, bright flashes of lightning and deafeningly loud claps of thunder. The area of Austin in which we live is called the hill country, and it's full of small canyons that do a great job of echoing sound when the lightning and thunder really get going.

The storms in life will come to and pass by all of us, but it's the attitude with which we endure the storm that determines the level of peace and joy we have while going through it.

As a storm would approach, Joker knew it and would begin to get nervous and bark at the door. So we'd let her in the garage, which had a comfy place to sleep by the door that goes into the house. As the booms of thunder and cracks of lightning would start, Joker would go nuts. She'd scratch at the wooden door, trying to get inside, shaking uncontrollably, whimpering and barking, until we let her in. Sam, on the other hand, would usually be close to the window, lying on his back with his paws in the air, sound asleep, occasionally snoring.

It struck me even then, as a child, how differently the two of them perceived the exact same situation. I noticed a few basic principles. One: The storm came to both of them. It made me think about how, in life, storms come to all of us. None of us are immune to them. Two: The storm ended for them both. Nearly all of the challenges in life have some kind of end. "This too shall pass." The final analysis is that the storms in life will come to and pass by all of us, but it's the attitude with which we endure the storm that determines the level of peace and joy we have while going through it.

Talking about storms reminds me of a very well-known story in the Bible that I learned in Sunday school while growing up. Jesus and the disciples are in a boat on the sea, and a huge storm pops up. The wind's blowing, the waves are high, it's raining, and probably even thundering and lightning. The disciples are looking at the storm (which is a key here), and they're scared stiff.

Freaking out, they go get Jesus who's in the cabin below, completely unconcerned about the storm above. Not only is He not worried but He's so at peace that He's asleep, maybe even snoring, like Sam the cat did. You see, Jesus realized that He had no need to be afraid and had an attitude of peace. He *knew* that God had a plan and that the storm would pass. His example tells us that our responsibility during the storms of life is to simply rest. Think about that. In the most challenging times in life, we should simply relax and trust God. How cool is that?

The disciples, meanwhile, were focusing their attention on the storm and created their own hysteria. Again, the storm affected all of them and ended for all of them. However, it was the disciples' worried attitudes and their focus through the storm that determined their overall lack of peace or unstable emotional "health."

WORRY

We have a lot of sayings in Texas. Some are deep and meaningful, and some are just plain silly, but there tends to be a little truth in all of 'em. When asked about how they feel about a particular situation, I've often heard people say, "I tried worryin', but it didn't do a bit a-good." Worrying about a storm in life will change absolutely nothing about the outcome.

However, worry *will* rob you of peace and sleep, increase your stress and blood pressure, create inflammation in your body, and turn you into someone nobody likes to be around. Many of you might be thinking right now, "I've tried not to worry so much, but I can't help it." If that's you, then there are a few questions you need to ask yourself: Are you an Ameri*can* or an Ameri*can't*? Just kiddin'. Seriously, you can help it, and you can change but you might need help. Many pieces of the health puzzle we've been referring to can affect your tendency to worry. In fact, worry will cause you to veer from your originally designed path—and there's a reason.

Spiritual health is a key in that God never intended for you to worry about anything—you weren't designed to. It's been His Original Design all along for you to "cast your cares" on Him, quite literally throwing them off of you and onto Him. It releases the pressure off of us. We aren't asked to share our troubles and doubts, insecurities and fears, but to throw them or "chuck 'em" as far from us as possible. When you understand this, it means that you know that if it's an issue that you can't change, letting it go and giving it to Him removes all responsibility from you and totally changes your attitude.

Imagine this scenario for a moment. You find out one day that the whole planet and the life of everyone living on it is dependent on *you* to solve a nearly impossible problem, which you can't possibly get done in any given period of time—not even in a million years. As you sit there, in despair, with the weight of the reality of your inability to handle it weighing you down, along comes someone to help you.

This person says, "Hi there, I'll solve this problem for you, no charge, and you get to go rest and relax by the pool—in total peace—while I do it. No strings attached. Oh, and by the way, I'm perfectly equipped to handle this issue (unlike you). I wrote the book on how to fix this problem, and I'll do a fantastic job, guaranteed. By the way, I love you very much!"

Can you imagine the sense of relief you'd feel and the attitude change? Talk about the weight of the world being lifted from your shoulders! But this is exactly what God does for us. He takes our worries away and simply says, "I'll handle it!" That's part of the Original Design.

FOCUS

Several years back, I was having "one of those days." You know the kind I mean. I had received some really bad financial news, I'd forgotten to do something important for someone and subsequently let them down, had a crick in my neck from sleeping wrong, broke my sunglasses, had a zit the size of the Astrodome on my nose, and I was running late. I couldn't find a parking spot as I was driving around the Super-Mart, and I got a flat tire pulling in to the space I eventually found at the back of the parking lot. Let's just say I wasn't very happy and may have thought or mumbled some less than positive words to myself as I was walking into the store with a forehead-wrinkled, disgusted look on my face.

Upon entering the front of the store, there was a young lady, who was an employee, stacking something into a large pyramid-like display. All of a sudden, everything went in to really slow motion as I realized that she was walking with a severe limp, had one arm drawn up at her side that was lifeless, and she also had facial and spinal distortion. She then zeroed in directly on me, out of the dozen or so people walking into the store, and said with one of the most beautiful and genuine smiles I've ever seen, "Isn't life wonderful, sir?"

As I walked by her, fighting back the tears, I smiled and said, "Yes, it is." Then I walked right out the exit door on the other side of the storefront, and walked back to my car where I sat and cried for about a solid five minutes. As tears rolled down my cheeks, I asked God to forgive me for being so ungrateful, self-absorbed, for focusing on my own problems, and for having such a rotten attitude.

Being a manly man, I want you to promise not to tell anyone this story—it'll ruin my in-control, confident, tough exterior. Just wait—there are more sappy stories later too. The point of this story is obvious, though. There I was with everything in the world going my way, save a few minor details, and I was sulking, plainly visible to everyone, with a stink face, and grumbling to myself. What right did I have to have an attitude like this at all, much less in a public place? The answer is: I didn't.

Now for a little justifying (don't you just love human nature?). I did actually have some challenges in that day that could understandably cause me to feel frustrated, but they didn't amount to much in the big scheme of things. I was putting my focus in the wrong place. Humans do this, though, don't we? Scientists who study driving call it "target fixation." Have you ever noticed that when you're in your car and you see something that catches your eye, you tend to steer toward it? Our whole body tends to move mentally and physically toward what we focus on. What are you focusing on?

We have to focus on the stable and unmoving nature of God and His Original Design to help us regain our health.

Here's another way of looking at it. What if I was doing my best Colonel Sanders impression and I was wearing a white three-piece suit, complete with white shirt, white socks, white shoes, and a white handkerchief. If there was a tiny red ink stain on my lapel about the size of a dime, what would your eyes be immediately drawn to when you saw me? The ink stain, of course. (I know you were thinking about my boyish good looks, but go with me for a moment.) Our brains instantly direct our eyes to the flaw, what's out of place, or the thing that's different than everything around it. Then we focus on that flaw and lose sight of the fact that every other inch of that suit is bright white and as clean as a whistle.

When you're out on a boat in the ocean and the waves are high and you're feeling seasick, what does the captain tell you to focus on? He'll tell you to look at the horizon because it's stable and unmoving. We've got to do the same thing with times of fear and doubt in our lives. We have to focus on the stable and unmoving nature of God and His Original Design to help us regain our health.

What if I walked up to you one day and said, "You know, I sure do think you're a great person. I want to give you this brick of 99.9% pure gold." Would you begin to whine and moan about the fact that 0.1% of it was not gold or even go so far as to throw it back at me, disgusted? Survey says…no way! You'd probably say, "Thank you!" and run to the bank as fast as you could while laughing and smiling and calling everyone you know to tell them how lucky you were. If you really think about it, haven't we been given a life that is 99.9% pure gold?

You can't immediately say, "No, my life stinks cuz I can't find a job." Or, "Life stinks cuz my booty don't fit in my jeans no more." All kidding aside, even if you've been dealt a serious blow like cancer or the loss of a loved one, you must keep your eyes focused not on the things that are going wrong, the things that you don't have, or the things that you haven't done. We all need to stay focused on all the good things that we're thankful for and have been given without deserving them in the least little way.

I call this taking "good inventory." When I'm feeling down or discouraged, I make a choice to ignore the noise and I take inventory of all the good things in my life. I remind myself of my blessings to put my focus back where it belongs.

About two years ago, one of my daughters was having a tough time and said, "Daddy, today was a bad day. I forgot my pencil, nobody played with me at the playground, I scraped my knee, and now I can't find my toy dog." She was really upset and actually shed a little tear. To her, it was a really big deal. I comforted her first, and then said, "What if we thought about all of the good things in your day…like you got to wear that beautiful dress, you had a yummy breakfast, you got to go on a field trip at school, and we're going to the park in a few minutes!" Her eyes lit up, she started smiling and even laughed a little. Just a simple repositioning of the mind set on the positive and she was in good shape!

We all need to live with an "attitude of gratitude" where we seek out and focus on the positive and beautiful things in our lives. Knowing how blessed we truly are, all things considered, shouldn't we be happy most of the time, while spreading joy to all of those whom we come into contact with? Having an attitude of gratitude has a way of blocking out the negativity that is trying to filter into your mind and ruin your life. You can't ever see the beauty of this world if you have your face down in the dirt.

As I'll talk about in the chapter on alignment, your actual posture should reflect the mental and spiritual "postures" in your life. By that I mean that when you have your head down, you have your neck bent down too, which distorts your normal posture and causes significant pain and damage to your spine over time. Similarly, when our "mental posture" is down by focusing on our problems and feeling sad or mad or sorry for ourselves, we're "hanging our heads" and living in a state of pain that can cause serious damage to our normal, healthy mental state. Remember the phrase, "Keep your chin up!"? It's true—quite literally.

When we keep our "spiritual posture" focused on our issues, we're "looking down" instead of looking up to God for guidance and help. When we have the right attitude and we point our focus upward, all of the pillars of health benefit as a result. That's part of the Original Design, too!

There's a principle here that really intrigues and motivates me. The principle is that what you focus on affects your life. To focus simply means to devote your mind and heart to only one thing…ignoring all else. If you spend five minutes in prayer, meditation on good things, laughing with family or friends, learning something that improves your life or any other positive thing, then that's five minutes of your waking hours that you *can't* spend being depressed or angry or frustrated at yourself or the world. You crowd out the bad with good. They can't both exist at the same time. I love that concept!

On the flip side, the more time you spend with negative people, or with negative thoughts, activities, and things that cause you to get frustrated or angry or stressed out, then that blocks out time you would've had to focus on positive, uplifting things. Not only does this limit the time that your mind will be in a good place, but it begins to shape the way you think and how you view yourself, others, and the world around you.

Your mind is a fragile and easily influenced machine that needs to be carefully guarded. We, like computers, are input/output beings that can be easily molded. We all know stories of kids who were told they were no good or that they would never amount to anything. Then, as they grew, they began to believe it and embodied what they heard until there was no difference between what started as a lie suggested to them and the reality of who and what they became. Their beliefs began to determine their actions. We're all like this.

It's like telling a lie so many times that you begin to eventually remember it and believe it to be something real that actually happened. Let's reverse that phenomenon by saying and thinking about positive things we want to see happen. After a while, they'll become reality to us. Our perception of the world around us is critical in determining how we think, how we feel, how we act, what we say, and, in the end, who we are. The only way to change our perception is to change our attitude by focusing on the good in our lives, and having a heart full of thanks.

CHAPTER 4

EMOTIONS

The words "emotional" and "mental" are often confused or interchanged with each other. Both are intangible and difficult to measure, but I'd say that "mental" is a broader category of the mind, based on thoughts and knowledge, whereas "emotional" is more of an outward effect, based on feelings. Nonetheless, you can't really objectively gauge how much emotional stress you have in your life.

There's no physical test that measures your emotions with a number, like your "normal" cholesterol number. No doctor or lab tech is going to tell you, "Well, the normal range for your emotional enzymes is between 100–150, and your number tested out to be 882!" This is because we can't isolate anything in the body that tells us how we're doing emotionally. However, most of us can "feel" when our emotions are out of whack. We just don't feel good about life and we know something is wrong. We often call it being "stressed." *Too* much bad stress can absolutely destroy health.

While not extremely scientific, we can get a rough estimate of our stress level with my "stress test" below. Answer with a scale of 0–10, with 0 being no stress at all and 10 is maximum stress:

1. When you think of your job, boss, and coworkers, what's your stress level?

2. When you think of your relationship with your spouse, what's your stress level?

3. When you think of your relationships with friends, what's your stress level?

4. When you think of your relationship with your family, what's your stress level?

5. When you think of your relationship with your kids, what's your stress level?

6. When you think of your time commitments to various obligations, what's your stress level?

7. When you think of your body self-image, what's your stress level?

8. When you think of your spiritual health, what's your stress level?

9. When you think of your ability to get sleep, what's your stress level?

10. When you think of your ability to get things accomplished, what's your stress level?

11. When you think of your ability to get exercise, what's your stress level?

12. When you think of your ability to eat a healthy diet, what's your stress level?

13. When you think of your financial status, what's your stress level?

14. When you think of your ability to take vacations or relax, what's your stress level?

15. When you think of how close you are to your purpose in life, what's your stress level?

Add up your score from each question to gauge your emotional health and find your "stress level." If your score is:

- 0–30, you have amazing emotional health. (You're in good shape and healthy.)

- 31–60, you have really good emotional health. (You're doing okay, but there's room for improvement.)

- 61–90, you have average emotional health. (This is not so good, so start working on it.)

- 91–120, you have poor emotional health. (You should actively pursue better emotional health.)

- 121–150, you have dangerously bad emotional health. (It's time to get professional help—now!)

Anything under stress, over time, will eventually break.

Getting a good idea of our stress level can help us determine whether or not we need to change some emotional stressors in our lives. Nearly anyone can handle a little stress for a short time, but all of us will begin to have major issues if our stress stays too high for too long. Anything under stress, over time, will eventually break.

All people will be affected differently by similar challenges that they may encounter, so emotional stress is truly based on how it affects that person specifically. Like so many things in the Original Design, it's unique to you. It's totally subjective and it only matters how *you* feel.

Emotion is incredibly powerful. My dad always says, "A man convinced against his will remains unconvinced still." He also says, "When emotion and reason are fighting inside someone's mind, emotion wins every time." What someone feels on the inside is extremely hard to change, and trying to change them with an argument is a waste of time. People change by an experience or situation that stirs their emotions at a deep level.

LETTING GO OF THE PAST

One of the big areas of emotional anguish for many people is the inability to let go of past events. If it's something that someone has done to us, we need to forgive them and move past it. Not forgiving will only create problems for our own health. In fact, they've probably already forgotten about it, but it's still hurting *us* on the inside. Holding on to hate is like drinking poison and expecting the other person to die.

All of us have had bad things happen, but we also have things in our lives that we regret doing or would've done differently knowing what we know now. Some might say, "I wouldn't change a thing," but I think if they were being completely honest, there is something they wish they hadn't said or done. Everyone has a little dark spot in their past, but some have what they, at least, would consider to be a huge dark spot. Some of you might even say that you've had multiple dark times or that you're in the dark right now.

Regardless of how you view it, the past is just that—in the past. So how do we move forward? I heard a very smart guy (Pastor Rob Koke) once say that you start out each day with just two things: the knowledge of the experiences that you had in the past and the faith for what is to come in the future. He was wrong, of course, because I also start the day with prayer, exercise, a nutritious breakfast, and I put my pants on—except for some Saturdays. Just kidding.

Seriously, all of us have been shaped by the experiences that we've had in our lives. Every time you encounter a situation where you have to make a decision, you go back into the "database" of your mind and quickly recall the necessary information to help you make a decision based on that knowledge. The trick is to keep the knowledge, but let go of the hurt.

A simple example that comes to mind is from just a few years ago. I told my youngest daughter, who was three at the time, not to touch the stove because it was extremely hot. I looked away for a second, and sure enough, she touched the stove and lightly burned her finger. Only a few days later, we were in the same situation and I again told her not to touch the stove. This time, I could see her pause and think about it as she reached her hand toward the stove. She thought for a few seconds, and then withdrew her hand. The information about what happened when she touched it was stored in her mind. She didn't cry again, she just retrieved the data.

We'd like to think that we can learn from the information were told by trusted people in our lives or experts in a particular field, and many times we do. But sometimes we just have to learn on our own. Either way, once that information is stored in our brains, we have nearly instant recall to use that information any time we need it.

The challenge is that we don't always make the correct decision based on what we know is right. We often base our decision on emotional factors. So if we truly want to change the way that we're living our lives to be more healthy, then we have to gain knowledge *and* change our emotions.

How many times in your life have you done something that you know, beyond a shadow of a doubt, was the wrong thing to do, but you still did it anyway? I think most of us would say we do those kinds of things all the time. So how do we change our behavior?

I've interviewed many of my friends and patients about what "clicked" in their heads when they finally made the changes that turned their health around. They almost always said that it was an accumulation of factors that mounted to a tipping point and/or one single event that changed something in their brains. They went from, "I really want to lose weight," to "I'm going to lose weight." For others, it was shifting from saying, "I'd like to start working out," to "I will start working out." The brother of one of my patients explained his "moment" like this:

> I'd been gaining weight for a long time, and my health problems were beginning to mount. By this point, I was over a hundred pounds overweight and was miserable. I was in pain all the time, had trouble moving around to do even normal activities of daily living, and really saw no point in living anymore.

He continued:

> I had an appointment at my doctor's office to get yet another medication added to the long list I already had, and was asked to have a seat in the waiting room. As I sat down on the chair, I crushed it, and broke one of the legs completely off of it as I fell onto the floor.

> Of course, people rushed to my aid, and as I laid there, the only thing that came to my mind was the question, "How did I let it get this far?" I decided right then and there that I was not going to spend another year in this downward spiraling health mess that I had started all by myself.

He had an incredibly powerful emotional moment that went to his core. What's the rest of his story? He went to the doctor to talk about lap band surgery to "shrink" the size of his stomach with surgical intervention. The doctor told him that because of how overweight he was and how high his blood pressure was he'd have to lose some weight before they could safely do the surgery. When he asked the doctor how to do this, the doctor told him that he'd have to start cutting calories and do some exercise. He answered with a confused look on his face, "Wait. So you're saying that you want me to diet and exercise?"

They both laughed and it dawned on him that what he needed to do was what he already knew to do all along but had never had enough motivation. Now the motivation was there because that emotional "click" happened in his brain. So he began to change his diet, eat less, exercise, and stretch, and within a year and a half he lost the weight without having a risky surgery.

FEAR AND REWARD

It's been said that people change due to one of two emotional circumstances: fear or reward. Everyone reacts differently and is more motivated by one or the other, but either way they're powerful in their ability to cause us to take action. Let me share a few stories to illustrate this point.

JESSICA'S STORY

I have a sweet patient who worked at a health-food store chain. She told me about a program they had for employees which specified that if you ate right and exercised enough to get your health scores (like blood work and body mass index) within certain guidelines, you'd receive a greater employee discount on your own grocery purchases. The better your "scores," the greater your discount.

She was excited about this opportunity and worked hard to reach this goal, even doing the 21-day purification program that we recommended for her. She drastically changed her diet and chose more organic whole fruits and vegetables and clean sources of protein. She also kicked up her exercise and stretching routine so that she was burning more calories, gaining strength, and slimming down. This caused her to sweat more frequently, which cleared her pores or sweat glands and helped her body detoxify.

After many weeks of working on it, she achieved her goal and met the requirements of the program. We were proud of her, and she was healthy, happy, and excited about getting her discount. She is one of those people who responded to the emotion of reward and responded to get the "prize" set before her, which also greatly improved her life.

MEARA'S STORY

Another dear patient of mine whom I knew from our church had come to me over the course of many years for various injuries or car accidents. We had candid conversations over the years about nutrition and exercise as she struggled with her weight, energy, self-image, and emotional health. Nearly every time she was in my office, we would discuss healthy eating habits and exercise. As the years passed, she "tried" multiple diets and exercise fads, she bought books and multiple resources to help her make positive changes to her health. Guess how much change she actually made over those years? You guessed it—none. Nothing changed. Meara had great intentions and daily felt the pain of what she saw in the mirror, the pain of her joints that were inflamed and fatigued from the added weight, and the pain of being tired all of the time and not being able to do what she knew she was called to do.

Eventually, she moved out of state and I didn't see her for several years. One day while seeing patients in my office, I came out to the lobby to greet a new patient, when I saw this beautiful, fit, healthy-looking lady who somewhat resembled Meara. She smiled at me and I smiled at her, and as I went back to my office, it dawned on me who she was. I came right back out to the front and said, "Meara! How are you? You look amazing!" A little later, we had a chance to chat, and, of course, I asked her, "What did you do?"

Here's her story in her own words:

> Three decades of yo-yo dieting and a lack of self-esteem left me hopeless and searching for a solution to my issue of being more than 100 pounds overweight. After numerous conversations with you, Dr. Mark, I recognized the truth that eating less and

moving more would be the simplest solution, but I didn't think or believe that plan would work for me.

When a health crisis and near-death experience occurred six years ago, I realized that time is precious and life is more limited than we think. So I chose to make changes that would serve me for the rest of my life. First, I had to decide to cut off all other options. I then realized that you have to make daily choices, moment by moment, to ensure the success of your decision. Last, I realized that discipline is remembering what you ultimately want! To be healthy, fit, and trim enables you to live life to the fullest!

She then told me about a conversation with her MD who told her how lucky she was to be alive and that her options were plain and simple. Option 1: She could continue living as she had and die young. Option 2: She could change her lifestyle and live. Wow. That's pretty scary and invokes a great deal of the emotion of fear. However, it was the fear of dying that deeply affected her and gave her the motivation *she* needed to change her life for the better.

THE MIND-BODY CONNECTION

People will often say, "Ah, it's all in your head!" Unfortunately, even some doctors will say this to their patients after they tell them about a health problem or something that's deeply affecting them. For a while, it was popular to say that something was psychosomatic when referring to a problem that one was just making up.

That's always been kind of funny to me since studying the mind-body connection in neurology class. The actual psychosomatic principle says that there is a response in the "soma," or body, to something initiated in the "psycho," or brain. Basically, it describes how a thought or emotion can create a change in your physiology.

Emotions are intangible but their effects on us *are* tangible.

For instance, if you get a phone call that someone you love has suddenly died, you might experience certain negative physiological changes like increased heart rate, blood pressure changes, nausea, vomiting, fainting, or even a heart attack. That doesn't sound like something that's *not* real to me. Just because I can't measure the emotion that triggered those reactions doesn't mean that it's not real. I can, however, measure the response to those emotions.

In fact, recent research confirmed that specific neural circuits and neurotransmitters respond to emotions and make measurable physiological changes.[1] Emotions do actually cause your body to function differently.

As humans, we're moved on a daily basis by emotions and feelings and things that we can't see or prove, but we feel them in our hearts and they're as real and powerful to us as any scientifically provable thing.

This shouldn't come as a surprise to any of us, because we often experience it on a daily basis. Think about going to lunch and your stomach growls. Think about something scary and you get goose bumps. Thoughts and emotions create physical reactions. Yes, emotions are intangible but their effects on us *are* tangible.

For instance, if someone tells you that you're fat, that will hurt you. You can't see or measure that emotional damage, but you then might eat more food because of the emotional stress that the words have caused in your life. Then, you can measure the amount of food you eat, your heart rate, cholesterol, blood pressure, waistline, and other factors that change as an end result of the actions you took after the comment that created a negative emotion.

"FAT BOY"

Remember the old phrase, "Sticks and stones may break my bones, but words will never hurt me"? Wrong. They're potentially *more* harmful than a physical wound! We're all emotional beings—yes, even the most macho, tough guys. What we think and feel affects our every action and word and internal function. We can't dismiss intangible emotions as having no impact on our lives. The mind's effect on the body is just as real as anything physical.

When I was about 13, I had put on a good deal of weight and was chunky. My nickname at the time was "fat boy." I knew I was overweight, but I wasn't sure how to change. Some of the joking was pretty emotionally damaging to me at the time. It was one of the lowest points of my life and a season where I had little self-esteem and things felt pretty hopeless. For years, I wouldn't let anyone see this picture:

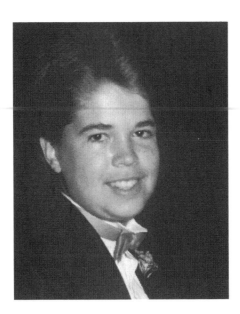

One time in particular that I'll never forget was when I was over at a friend's house and went swimming with two girls and two other guys. I was interested in one of the girls and had been for some time. They paired up in the pool and not only left me as the odd man out, but they began to gang up on me. The comments were harsh enough that I went home and angrily wrote a journal page with knife-stabbing pain in my heart and tears in my eyes. I found that note the other day, so here's a little bit from that (edited) entry:

> All they do is make fun of me and say, "Oh look, fat boy is getting his feelings hurt," and then they laugh! How do you think I feel being ridiculed for four days by their cut-downs, sarcasm, and rudeness!? I hear whispering, and then something about me being fat and then laughter again. I hate it so much!

Their words really hurt, but it was a turning point for me—it was the "click moment" in my brain, and I gave my heart to God that year. I also asked my dad what I needed to do to get in shape, and he told me about the kind and amount of junky food that I was eating. Then he taught me how to work out and be active and make choices that improved my health.

By my senior year in high school, I got in great physical condition, I was involved in my youth group at church, got elected senior class president and student council vice president, had a great girlfriend, and was voted prom king. I had finally gotten to a place of peace and health on many levels.

Sometimes the toughest emotional challenges can cause us to make changes that shape the rest of our lives. None of us like the pain of emotional hurt, but we can't let it hold us back. Those wounds can either destroy us or propel us forward toward our Original Design. We get to choose. Why not choose to let your low points become turning points?

TAKE EMOTIONAL INVENTORY

As with all of the chapters in this book, it's a good idea to take some time and sit down and be totally truthful with yourself about the subject of that particular chapter. In this case, take an "inventory" of your emotions and determine where the negative emotions in your life are coming from.

Is there a relationship (past or current) that's bringing you down? Is your job causing you to "blow your top"? Is your financial situation (debt, overspending, maxed-out credit cards) stressing you out? Whatever it is, write it down, pray about it, and determine if it's something that you can deal with on your own or if it requires professional help. Eliminating these negative emotions will be a significant key to achieving the optimal health that we all want and deserve.

Again, we also then need to take a "good inventory" of all the positive emotions in our lives and their roots. These are the things to recognize, reinforce, be thankful for, and focus on as sources of power, strength, and calming in our lives. These emotions bring joy and peace and happiness and are a true health jackpot. It's so important for our emotional health to be in balance if we're going to walk in our Original Design.

CHAPTER 5

REALITY AND CHANGE

It's often easy to read a health book or attend a health conference and get inspired and totally pumped up. If you're optimistic, you might think to yourself, "Wow, this is cool. I know I need to make some changes, and I'm gonna be the healthiest I've ever been! I can totally do this!" You may even start out doing really well and catch a mental glimpse of what the "new you" could actually look like.

Then reality sets in and you realize that it's hard, and it's a lot of work, because it's so different from what you've been doing. Habits have to change concerning when, how much, and where you eat; your budget allocation toward healthy food; time spent planning, preparing, cooking, and cleaning up after healthy meals; time spent exercising versus watching TV; and sleep changes. You may even realize that there are people or things you need to cut out of your life, and you begin to get discouraged. Even being optimistic, change is hard. Period.

However, stick with me, because there are some things that make it easier. The first step to getting out of a hole that you find yourself in is to put down your shovel. Many of us are creating our own issues and simply need to stop doing certain things…then we can move on to what we need to start doing.

The people who lean toward being a little pessimistic might be reading or listening to all the information in this book and thinking to themselves something like, "Yeah, sure! Dr. Mark is crazy if he thinks that I'm going to be able to do all of the things that he's suggesting in this book. It would absolutely take me the rest of my life to change or accomplish even half of the things he's asking me to!" I get it. I hear you.

**The first step to getting out of a hole that
you find yourself in is to put down your shovel.**

I've often felt the same way when reading other people's books, but I'm a realist and an opportunist, which is somewhere smack in the middle of being an optimist and a pessimist. You can't allow yourself to get "paralysis by analysis" and go to the extreme of doing nothing simply because it seems too hard. You have to take action and grab the opportunity to get healthier—just be realistic about it! You also can't allow yourself to burn out and give up because you tried making too many changes all at once. You've got to be realistic and accept that this is going to take a while to become who you were designed to be, but you have to actually start.

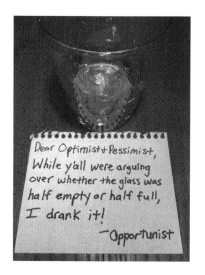

Most of us are pretty off-track—some of us more than others. We can *all* make changes, but we can't be perfect all the time. Let's not get hung up on the fact that we ate one little thing that was unhealthy or that we didn't exercise for a week or we didn't get enough sleep for days on end. I don't know anyone who's perfect all the time. We all miss the mark, but often not by as much as we think.

Don't let messing up get you down!

"BROADWAY JOE"

One of the greatest, most successful and loved quarterbacks of all time in the NFL was Joe Namath, nicknamed "Broadway Joe" after being on the cover of multiple magazines. His career pass completion average was 50.1%. The reality is that he missed his target nearly exactly half of the time! Think about that for a second. He was one of the most talented and elite players of all time, and he failed as much as he succeeded. Your average, professional, "cream of the crop" NFL quarterback does much less than that. Don't let messing up get you down!

If you don't achieve perfection in any area of health, it's because you're human and we all fail every now and then—even the best of us. Joe was a highly trained professional. Hardly any of us have been trained how to be healthy *at all*, so we can't be too hard on ourselves.

How can we expect to succeed in being healthy if all we've ever known is what we saw Mom and Dad or friends do? Proper training and regular practice are the keys to becoming really good at something—including being healthy! In fact, I'd say that many, if not most, of us have been trained by marketing companies that want us to believe that "fruity hoops" are "a part of this nutritious breakfast." Yeah, the *not* nutritious part. Are marketing companies more concerned with your health or their profits? They don't love you; they love your money! We have to analyze where we're getting our "training" from on how to achieve health. It's critical to our success.

Hopefully this book is the beginning of a long journey that will train you to achieve an elite level of health. You need to know that when you mess up, which we all do at times, it's just not that big of a deal! Move on and make a better decision next time. We have to accept the reality that change is challenging and will require a learning curve over a period of time. After that, it gets much easier and only takes a small amount of fine-tuning as we go through life. Like Joe, it's about good training, consistency, and striving to be the best we can be! It's not about being perfect all the time—we need to loosen up and have fun!

BE REALISTIC

I think we should be realistic about what changes we can make right now and take those steps first. For instance, let's say that you'd like to prepare a healthy meal for your family. Then reality sets in and you realize that you've got three more errands to run before you pick up the kids at ballet or baseball practice, and you have very little time left. Normally you'd just say, "Well, there just isn't enough time in the day to do everything that I need and want to do, so I guess we'll just stop at the fried-chicken joint and pick up a nugget family pack."

What I'd ideally encourage you to do is to take out a little bit of time at the beginning of the week to plan meals and then you might have a healthy dinner in the crockpot or in the fridge all ready to go when you get home. A compromise, though, for the initial transition period to totally healthy choices might be to pick up the chicken, but go with grilled instead of fried, and skip the biscuits and fries and have a quick salad or veggie sticks with it at home.

In this way, you know you're making at least some better choices for you and your family, but you still stay on schedule and avoid eating late. Otherwise, you'd have to try to start cooking an entire healthy meal when you get home. Of course fast-food chicken is not ideal in the least, but again you're in transition and you've taken steps in the right direction. Do ya smell what I'm cookin'?

SOMETHIN' IS BETTER THAN NOTHIN'

Occasionally, my regular schedule gets derailed, which used to drive me nuts! It's like when I'm getting ready for work in the morning and have great intentions of working out only to look at the clock and reality sets in. I only have ten minutes before I need to be in the shower! Ahh! The obvious reaction is to be frustrated and just blow off the workout altogether, and frankly that's exactly what I used to do. This would set my entire day off on a really bad foot.

Well, one day (in a little bit of anger) I went downstairs to exercise for ten minutes anyway, because, "Dang it! I'm not about to miss another stinkin' workout!" When I did, I had an epiphany. Doing something, even though it was less than I wanted to do, was still a positive action and led to me feeling better about myself. In the end, that little workout gave me a nice little muscle pump, a good emotional release, and some added energy as well. I wasn't nearly as disappointed in myself, and the day went much better overall!

You could apply this to nearly any area of your life. No time to get a card for that special person's birthday? No big deal. Get a sticky note and jot down a quick note to them with something you love or admire about them. Just show some effort from the heart. They'll be more touched than you might imagine and may even appreciate it more than just a signed store-bought card. I know *I would*.

Maybe you've heard me speak before about naps and you've vowed to get that 20-minute nap in, but the day was crazy and you have five minutes left during your "nap window." It's okay because that's reality! Get still, close your eyes, and just shut down and rest for those five minutes. It'll still make a significant difference and you won't feel defeated. There's a little moral victory there that will inspire you to try again the next day.

Here's another scenario. Plan A: You may normally say, "I'm too darn tired to exercise!" and so you flop down on the couch at the end of your day with a tub of ice cream and begin to watch several hours of mind-melting junk on TV. Plan B: When you get home from work, I'd encourage you to eat a light, healthy meal to get some energy, and then drink some water. Rest quietly with your eyes closed for up to 20 minutes and then get 20–30 minutes of light exercise in before watching a little TV. I promise you'll feel much better physically and much better about yourself than if you'd done plan A.

Does plan B sound laughable to you? Instead of being discouraged and thinking you can't and wouldn't do what I'm suggesting and just blowing it off, try a transitional compromise. Plan C: Have a snack and rest while you watch a half hour of mind-empowering or relaxing TV, then do some push-ups, squats, or stretches while you watch another half hour of TV. Finding the middle ground in the beginning transitional period between the "old you" and the "new you" might be just the encouragement you need to realize that you can do it.

In any area of health, doing what you can is important. If you just can't fit it all in, that's okay. Do what you can joyfully and without regret. Later, take some time to reevaluate your priorities and plan to make a few changes where they're needed.

PLAN AHEAD

It's a great idea to plan ahead for meals, exercise, sleep, and otherwise prioritize other areas that you know are important for your health and your family's health. At first it seems like a lot of work to plan ahead, but then you find it actually frees up quite a bit of time and eliminates a good deal of stress.

For instance, if you plan ahead to have healthy snacks at home, at the office, or in the car for the kids when they get hungry, then you won't be tempted to get something junky from the vending machine or the fast-food place that'll make you feel guilty and hurt your health. The reality is that if you don't plan ahead, you probably aren't going to get much change. If you do start planning ahead, however, you'll be well on your way, having already made these little changes, and you'll have some confidence to make even more.

NHE

I'd like to introduce a concept that's useful to understanding or evaluating any activity, event, or action, as to whether or not it's of value to your overall health. The reality is that, in the end, not all things are beneficial to your health. Even things that seem to be a good idea in the beginning may prove to be a bad idea after some careful evaluation. The concept is something I call the Net Health Effect, or "NHE."

This can be an important idea to consider when people try to improve their health, only to become sicker in the process. NHE is determined by evaluating all of the factors surrounding a particular action, behavior, or relationship.

For example, many would agree that jogging is healthy. However, consider jogging on concrete, down the side of the interstate, in beat-up old sneakers, in 105-degree heat, with bad posture, while inhaling exhaust fumes and enduring all the pounding to the joints of the feet, ankles, knees, hips, and spine. You could easily argue that the benefits of jogging, in *that* way, are outweighed by the negative repercussions of how it's done.

This goes back to the idea of balance that we discussed earlier. We have to reach our goal of optimal health by considering all of the pillars of health instead of just focusing on one aspect of the situation.

Here's another angle. Many people would say that being in a dating relationship is a good thing, right? Ah, it's spring, love is in the air, and you're diving headlong into a romance with someone exciting and new. Time goes by and you're now madly and passionately in love with that person. Well, the challenge would be that if you discovered over time that this person didn't share many of your values, was a bad influence on you in relation to diet, exercise, drug or alcohol use, didn't respect you, didn't encourage you, was abusive in some way, and otherwise created a great deal of stress in your life. The side effects of *that* relationship could include anger, guilt, frustration, insomnia, excessive weight gain or loss, lung or liver damage, sadness, fear, insecurity, depression, going to prison, or even suicide, just to name a few.

The NHE of that relationship would definitely be negative. You might want to strongly consider finding a different relationship with more positives and less negatives—a relationship that has side effects of joy, strength, a positive self-image, respect, laughter, peace, security, success, and health.

How does one determine the NHE of something? Well, it's very simple. Make a pros and cons list. You list each positive and negative aspect of the activity or person in question, and then compare your two columns. If there's a clear predominance of negative aspects, then it might be something that does not help you in your overall goal of achieving optimal health. As you might guess, it's not perfectly mathematical, though. Your pros column for something may be longer but a few of the con items on the list are so bad that you clearly need to cut it completely out of your life.

On the flip side, something you're evaluating the NHE of may have a long cons list, but they are relatively minor in total when compared to the few but amazing items on the pros list. In the end, I think we all know what's right in our hearts and whether or not it adheres to the Original Design for our lives. Prayer and seeking the wise counsel of mentors and people you trust is also a good way to help evaluate the NHE of something.

DO IT NOW

None of us like change, right? Going through this process can be a little difficult or painful. However, it's far better to go through the mild to moderate pain of making changes now than to have a negative obstacle in your life that creates an unbelievably huge amount of pain later. At that point, there's a ton of damage that you absolutely have to change just to survive. In that state, you might be so tired and beat-up that it's extremely hard to change or there's even irreparable damage that you can't change or reverse. You can't go back.

The time to face reality and make the change is now! Make the change *before* the damage occurs. So many doctors talk about "early detection." It's commonly discussed as one of the most critical factors in staying healthy. I'd agree, but what about living in such a way as to prevent problems in the first place?

Prevention is a much better way to go. For instance, do you skip brushing and visit the dentist only to detect cavities, or do you brush your teeth in order to prevent them? The problems associated with not taking action now could apply to so many different aspects of health. Many times I talk to patients who say, "I just wish I would've done something sooner! I knew better, but I just didn't do anything about it." This doesn't have to be you!

We could be talking about a spinal or extremity (knee, elbow, wrist, etc.) misalignment that was creating pain and dysfunction for years, but sadly the pain was ignored for too long and permanent damage occurred. What are the most common words heard in a chiropractic office? "I thought it would go away."

When someone has a poor overall pattern of eating, it may simply cause them to feel bad or be low on energy at first. However, over time, it's common that those poor habits directly contribute to cardiovascular disease, diabetes, obesity, cancer, and a host of other serious health issues. We all know how many of these diseases end up if they are allowed to continue without eliminating the source of the problem early on in the process.

You get the idea. The list goes on and on, but the same is true for all of them. They all involve continuing to do something that we know isn't healthy but we keep doing it anyway. We need to make the changes now to prevent the problems from ever occurring in the first place. There could be many reasons why we're continuing these things. It may be that we're scared to make a change, unsure of what to change, comfortable (lazy) in the situation, or simply unaware that we're being affected negatively by something or someone.

Proverbs reminds us: "For the waywardness of the simple will kill them, and the complacency of fools will destroy them; but whoever listens to me will live in safety and be at ease, without fear of harm" (Proverbs 1:32-33 NIV). As I see it, "waywardness…kills" means that veering from the Original Design will harm you, "complacency" is choosing not to take action steps to change, "listens to me" is listening to wisdom and following what He put in your heart, and to "be at ease" means a state of ease or health that is the opposite of dis-ease.

Regardless of the reason, facing the reality of the situation, making a change, and doing it now is critical. It's the only thing that will get us off of the wrong track that's headed in the wrong direction, and back on the right track, headed in the right direction. The right track is simple. It is and always will be the Original Design for our lives.

YOUR CHANGE IS UNIQUE TO YOU

You cannot buy into the lie that there is no right and wrong, that no one thing is better than another, and that all things are relatively equal. That's simply not true. Nearly every area of your life *does* have an ideal state that's unique to you. There are foods that are better for you than others. There are ways to exercise that are more beneficial than others. There is an alignment of your body that's the most ideal. There is a relationship and strategy to maintaining that relationship that's better than another. There is an amount of sleep that's better for you. You *can* change toward that ideal! Don't give up just because it's been one way for so long.

ROSS'S STORY

One of my favorite stories is about a super nice patient of mine named Ross. When he first came in, he was sitting with his arms crossed, skeptical and quiet. His wife was coming in for an initial evaluation after they moved to Austin from another state where she'd been seeing a chiropractor for decades. He had an injury 30 years before and had given up on the possibility of change. When it happened, he had tried "everything" to get past the right upper back and neck pain, ringing in both ears, and hearing loss in the right ear, but nothing changed with traditional treatments. He had tried multiple medications and therapies from "more doctors than I could count," he would say.

As I always try to do, I began to talk to him and find some common ground. Eventually we hit it off, he began to open up, and agreed to try chiropractic. We did an exam and took X-rays and found multiple misalignments in his upper cervical spine. After one adjustment, he noticed a difference in the ringing in his ears, and by 12 visits he had nearly no ringing or hearing loss at all! With tears in his eyes, he gave me a big hug and said, "I can hear a clock ticking across the room for the first time in 30 years!"

Since it'd been so long since his issues began, it would've been easy to assume that there was no way anything could ever change, and to just give up. In fact, he *had* given up, but he decided to try just one more time. I'm sure glad he did, and I know he was too.

You *can* change where you are.
You're *not* stuck. What you see in your life
now is not what it has to be in the future.

THINGS CAN CHANGE

One additional point to keep in mind is that your ideals in each area can and may very likely change throughout the course of your life. What you're looking for in a dating relationship may change from when you're 17 to when you're 37. The amount of sleep you need will be different at 7 vs. 77, and so on. The seasons of life may change, but there's still an ideal that's specific to you.

Also, what's best for you may be (and probably will be) totally different than what is best for your friend, coworker, or family member. So don't "cheat off of their homework" and try to copy what someone else is doing. Do what you know is right, in your heart, for you. Believe you can change, ask God for help, and don't ever give up. You *can* change where you are. You're *not* stuck. What you see in your life now is not what it has to be in the future.

We've all heard that the definition of insanity is doing the same thing over and over again but expecting different results. It's so true. You'll never change unless you start doing things differently. It's also been said that the one thing that remains constant in life is change. It has to remain constant in our lives to achieve what's best, specifically, for us and for our families. Life is change. Life is motion. Life is flow.

Hey, I understand that we all have limitations and that we have to be realistic about change, but that doesn't mean settling for less than the best. Don't ever settle for less than what you know you were designed for. Things can change. Your path is unique and special and amazing. Remember, it's *your* Original Design.

CHAPTER 6

RELATIONSHIPS

Relationships are central to the human life and provide amazing health benefits in so many different ways. Most of us can cite at least one relationship that's extremely important to us. Whether it's your spouse, a parent, a sibling, a child, a friend, or a coworker, we all know someone we value tremendously and know that without that relationship our lives would be significantly less full. We need those relationships. Being alone all the time isn't fun and could in fact be dangerous.

When people are put in solitary confinement in prison, it's considered the worst form of punishment that can be given. Not only do they endure physical misery, but they can have permanent mental damage. In fact, only 5% of prisoners are in solitary confinement, but they make up 50% of the suicides in prison. That's no coincidence.

There's no doubt about it…your enemy wants you to be alone, separated from the safety of the pack. The Bible says, "It's not good for man to be alone" (see Genesis 2:18). It's important for like-minded people to come together in groups like churches, sports teams, special interest groups, and organizations of all kinds. There's a certain richness and stability in life that comes from sharing life with others that you just can't get by yourself.

My pastor says it like this: "When you get alone for too long, you can get weird!" Had the Unabomber had a friend, he might have told him, "You want to do what? That's ridiculous, dude! Let's go have lunch." You need people to keep you in check and to share life with.

Let's say you win the lottery. It's pretty darn exciting by itself, but what's the first thing that nearly anyone would want to do when they find out that they've won? They wanna call someone, scream, and share what happened! That allows them to multiply their joy immediately by experiencing the excitement all over again. That's not random; it's part of the Original Design.

My daughters are always doing something cute. Wait. Guess what? One of my daughters just now came in to my study (as I was writing this) and randomly typed this on my keyboard about two paragraphs down: "I love daddy." How can I delete that? I moved it to this paragraph. I think it fits pretty well right here. Wow. Priceless! That actually just happened.

Sorry. Anyway, they'll do something like a little dance or a drawing with crayons and then they'll turn to me and say, "Daddy, look what I can do!" or "Look what I did!" I, of course, get really excited and say, "Wow, sweetie! That's awesome!" or "That's beautiful!" They smile and glow with joy to get positive affirmation and usually want a hug. It's one of the greatest mutual feelings there is.

They're excited to share something about their lives and *I'm* touched and thrilled to know that they want to share it and interact with me. It's a total win-win situation! Then, when I suggest that they go and show Mommy, they light up and squeal with excitement as they run down the hall to get to do the sharing and hugging all over again.

We're designed to share life with others. Tell your family, your friends, and tell God about your day. Share your dreams, your triumphs, and your failures. The greatest things in life are made even better by sharing with the ones we love, and the worst things are made easier by "getting it out" with them too.

The more meaningful relationships we have, the more joy we will have in our lives. But there's one relationship that tops them all—that's our relationship with God. We'll get into this relationship much more in the chapter on faith, but let's just say that it's the most fulfilling, meaningful, life-giving relationship we can have. Next to that relationship, the one with your spouse is of next greatest importance.

The one who elevates the anger, escalates the danger.

MARRIAGE RELATIONSHIPS

There's no doubt that one of the most important human relationships you can have is a marriage. There have been thousands of books written on the topic, so I'll leave most of it to the experts. However, there are a few tips that I'd like to share that have been beneficial for me and my beautiful, brilliant, funny, and amazing wife, Gabrielle. (Do I get points for saying that?)

Giving love, having it accepted, and then having it returned has got to be one of the greatest emotions that a person can feel in life. It does take all three components for a healthy marriage relationship. For example, if you give it, but it's not returned, then it feels empty. If you're in this kind of relationship, I strongly urge you to seek counseling and get to the root of the problem. There's often something that can be navigated through to get you past the issue and back to the kind of relationship that you were originally designed to experience.

Dealing with challenges in marriage relationships, or of any kind really, is difficult for all of us. It's human nature to want to strike out when we feel threatened or offended. Many times, our instant reaction is to trump the offensive words that the other person said to us with something even stronger. The one who elevates the anger, escalates the danger. The danger, of course, is that you'll say something you didn't actually mean that deeply hurts the other person, but now you can't take it back. Giving in to anger and hate will benefit no one.

Sometimes we're too self-centered or even just too lazy to really try to understand what the other person is feeling. We need to give our full focus to what their perception of the issue is and really, fully understand their side. It would be wise to treat it like someone who's giving you a detailed description to the location of hidden treasure. If you knew they *actually* had the directions, you'd pay close attention to every detail and you'd make sure you fully understood. The truth is that the hidden treasure of trust and love is waiting for those who take the time to listen and understand.

The grass isn't greener on the other side of the fence; it's greener where you water it!

Of course, my wife and I love each other, but we also have a mutual respect for each other, cheer the other on, have a huge measure of grace for each other, try to accept responsibility for doing something dumb, and ask for forgiveness when we do. These are all major keys to a healthy marriage relationship, but we discovered one other secret that I'd like to share. We always try to "out-serve" each other. When we see a way that we can help the other, we do our best to do it, even without them knowing we did it. It speaks volumes when we put the other person first, ahead of our own needs.

Patients will occasionally share with me that the flame is going out in their marriage and maybe that they've even begun seeking a new relationship. At the appropriate time and with love, I try to share with them that the grass isn't greener on the other side of the fence; it's greener where you water it! That new relationship will end up like the first one if they repeat the same mistakes they made before.

People have a tendency to stop "dating" each other when they get married. When dating, they're putting their best foot forward, getting all dressed up, shaved, smelling good, and acting as sweet and agreeable as they can be. They do thoughtful things for each other, buy gifts, say loving words, spend lots of time together, and have great physical intimacy. The perfect book describing this is called *The Five Love Languages* by Gary Chapman. If you haven't read it and your marriage is in crisis, then I'd encourage you to read it. It saved the marriage of some close friends of ours.

Within reason, we have to keep doing the things that we did when we were dating if we want to feel the same feelings that we had then. How we act toward each other is what generates those feelings of being "in love." If you took care of your body, dressed attractively, and did romantic things when dating and then stopped those things, that's kind of false advertising, isn't it? You essentially told him or her, "Hey, if you marry me, here's what you get!" Then after you got married, if you let yourself go, started wearing sweatpants to dinner, picking your nose and being disinterested, are you really surprised if your spouse begins to look elsewhere? Really?

We all love the excitement of the dating phase of a relationship—so keep it up. Think of all the things you used to do and re-create them on a regular basis. If you don't continue dating each other, either one or both of you may begin to seek that same excitement somewhere else. You *can* have it again; just make a decision to make new moments of excitement happen now and in the future.

There are many great books about the following subject, but I want to touch on something really quickly. An amazing woman I knew used to say that if a marriage was in trouble, it probably started in the bedroom. That wise lady was my grandmother!

Sex is an incredibly important part of a healthy marriage relationship and is a crucial part of the Original Design in so many ways. Your physical health even benefits from a healthy sex life. Please seek help if this is a problem in your marriage. It can be one of the greatest or worst parts of your relationship with your spouse.

In the end, marriage relationships are one of the most commonly cited reasons that people give when explaining what is creating the most stress in their lives or what gives them the biggest sense of security and joy. If you have kids, they need to know that their parents love each other just as much as they need to know that you love them. A solid marriage relationship is at the core of the state of emotional health for anyone who's married. Take the time and effort to keep the "home fires burnin'"!

DON'T DATE PEOPLE WITH "BIG BUTS"

Notice, that's not *butts* with two t's! No hate mail please. ☺ As with nearly anything, you have to create some relationship boundaries and limitations in several different ways. First off, you must create a huge boundary between you and damaging relationships.

I'm always amazed at patients or friends who are involved in dating relationships that are full of anger, violence, lying, distrust, disrespect, jealousy, or even just a lack of happiness and fun. It blows me away that they're willing to be involved in these relationships and even commit to marrying this person. What? Are you kidding me? If this is how the relationship is now, before marriage, then how do they think it will be after they get married? Getting hitched certainly doesn't make problems go away…it only magnifies them.

I always tell these people to watch out for "buts"—especially really big "buts"! If they say, "Well, he's a really good-looking guy, or a really wealthy guy, or a really funny guy, *but*…he's really mean or rude or dishonest or a bad influence on me," they should run. If there's a "but" included in the first sentence you think of to describe your significant other, then you might want to reconsider whether or not this is the right relationship for you, especially if it's a really big "but"! As I have two daughters, I may write a book about relationships and title it *Why You Should Never Date Guys with Big Buts!*

Hey, wait though, girls can have issues too. Some guys say, "She's really cute, but she yells at the top of her lungs every time I say hello to another female or forget to put the toilet seat down at her apartment." Perhaps she has some emotional challenges that need sorting out before you decide to spend the rest of your life with her. Girls can have big "buts" too!

Now don't get me wrong, I'm not a crazy head. There are obviously no perfect people, and anyone you marry or, more frankly, anyone you have a relationship with will have flaws. You have flaws. I have flaws—big ones. (Don't tell my wife—she hasn't noticed yet!) Seriously, though, we all do. However, while some of these flaws may be small and inconsequential to the overall health of the relationship, some may be huge red flags that tell you to get out now. You simply have to evaluate the NHE of a dating relationship to see whether or not it's healthy.

However, if you're in *any* relationship that routinely brings you down, causes you to be tempted to do things or say things you know you shouldn't, causes you physical or emotional harm, makes you cry, or sends your blood pressure skyrocketing, then you need to immediately work on getting away from that abuse—ASAP. There are no words that can fully explain just how toxic that bad relationships can be in our lives and to our overall health. It destroys who we are and who God designed us to be. We can't achieve ideal health or discover our purpose when living in the prison of a toxic relationship.

BAD BY-PRODUCTS

Depression is one by-product that is rampant among those who are or were in relationships associated with any of the emotions I discussed above. An alarming number of people feel so overwhelmed by depression that they seek out drugs to just help them function. In fact, antidepressants are the number-one class of prescribed medications.

In one study, the CDC looked at 2.4 billion drugs prescribed in visits to doctors and hospitals in 2005. Of those, 118 million were for antidepressants. "Depression is a major public health issue," said one doctor at Columbia University College of Physicians and Surgeons in New York City. When asked her opinion about the rapid rise in prescriptions for depression, she said, "The fact that people are getting the treatments they need is encouraging."[1] Wait? People living on drugs for the rest of their lives is "encouraging"?

I really do understand that, in certain circumstances, medication can be a temporarily useful and critically important tool. However, it's not and never will be part of anyone's Original Design to be on a drug forever. In getting medicated, many people are simply ignoring the underlying issue that often involves an unhealthy past or current relationship. It breaks my heart for them—they're in a drug prison that keeps them chained to the pain, which is only softened a little by the medication which may have other horrible consequences.

According to a report released by the National Center for Health Statistics, the rate of antidepressant use in the US, among teens and adults (people ages 12 and older) increased by almost 400% between 1988 and 2008![2] That's not okay. Nearly every single one of the mass shooting massacres in the news over the last 20 years involved a shooter on a psychotropic drug of some sort! (You **never** hear about this in the media—only more cries for gun control.) This is not the answer, people! We've got to get hearts healed and emotional and spiritual health restored.

Anger is another by-product of toxic relationships. When there's not a sufficient level of respect shown by someone that you're in a relationship with, there will many times be resentment and outright anger. It's often a result of being in a relationship that you know isn't right and it's causing your heart to feel unsettled and bitter, which in turn can cause you to do or say things that you might deeply regret later in life.

Frankly, the wrong relationships have a seemingly endless list of other bad by-products associated with them, like jealousy, fear, guilt, frustration, anxiety, anger, resentment, and high levels of stress which lead to indirect effects like overeating, heart and digestive issues, self-hate and illness. In the end, you simply waste your life not being in *good* relationships, and not being who you were designed to be.

CHOOSE YOUR FRIENDS CAREFULLY

Nearly every parent hopes and prays that their children make wise choices when it comes to the friends that they choose to hang out with. This is because parents know that the people we surround ourselves with, to a great degree, influence the person we become, or at least the way that we act when we're around them.

Show me a person's friends and I'll show you that person's future. Choosing friendships is extremely important in becoming who we were designed to be. We can't all be sports stars or brain surgeons, but we can all be the wonderful person God designed us to be. Friends can either push us closer to or further away from becoming that person. By the way, friends can have "big buts" too. ☺

I have a friend who, like many of us, wanted so badly to hang out with the cool people in high school that she went to nearly all the parties that involved drinking, drugs, and sexual misconduct. She, in fact, *was* a cool person, but she didn't think she was. She knew everyone and wanted to impress them, and many times that involved doing things she knew weren't right. We all have that still small voice that tells us when something that we're about to do is wrong.

Well, she started to get in trouble at school, in trouble with her parents, and, as we've all heard this story before, she became addicted to drugs and alcohol. It began at a very young age, maybe in sixth or seventh grade, and it all started with the friendships she chose.

Flash forward 25 years from high school and she's still stuck in that same rut, addicted to substances and leading a sad, depressed life, with only surface-level friendships. Her "friends" are not there for her, and they aren't trustworthy, loyal, caring, or sensitive to her needs. Many of them also bought in to the same lifestyle and now they're in the same boat and…it's not a party anymore.

We'll never become who we were designed to be when we chase the approval of others. We'll do increasingly stupid things to try to feel loved and accepted, when the only thing that will ever fill that void is a relationship with God and His love. When we receive the unconditional love of God, then we'll begin to see ourselves the way He sees us. That's who we were originally designed to be. We'll then love ourselves unconditionally and won't need the approval of others.

I've personally been blessed with a life that's full of friendships that are truly remarkable. I've also had quite a few relationships that I've had to end as well. It's hard to pick and choose, but you must be careful who you spend your time with. The Bible calls it "iron sharpening iron," or hanging out with people who make you a better person and get you closer to your originally designed purpose.

Sit down and set everything in your head aside—your past, your current situation, finances, health status, job, relationships, etc.—and simply ask yourself, "Who do I want to be ten years from now?" If your answer is different than the direction you're headed and different from who you are now, then one thing you need to do is evaluate your relationships. You need to prayerfully decide about each one, if you should continue pursuing growing it, or put it on the back burner, or just end it now.

If you aren't left with many relationships in the grow column after this analysis, then you need to start hanging around people you want to be like. But let's not become stalkers—there are appropriate and inappropriate ways to do it. If you really want to be like the president, I'd expect it would *not* be wise for you to move to Washington, DC, jump the fence at the capitol, and yell, "Hi! I wanna be like you! Can we hang out?"

Right idea, wrong action. A natural connection will take place with those you're designed to be around. You won't have to beg them; they'll want to be around you too. Let it happen naturally. Don't force it.

One way to be like a public figure whom you admire is to read the books they've written, watch the speeches they've done, or study the things that they do. Books, CDs, videos, and podcasts are a great way to "pick someone's brain" without physically hanging out with them. Once you've learned a great deal about them, then think about the ways that you're different, and begin taking steps toward what you admire about them.

It's still important to pick people to be close to in the normal day-to-day world you admire, who encourage and inspire you, who you see treat others the way you would like to, or who generally are more like who you'd like to be. That's why I hang out with my wife as much as I do. (More points?)

At work, at school, in church, or in your community, find a person or two and plant some seeds. Ask them if they'd like to have lunch or coffee or hang out some time. Tell them you really appreciated how they handled this situation, or how they handled that relationship. Explain that you're trying to become the best person you can be and you see some attributes in them that you admire and would like to emulate. Remember, not everyone is looking for a new friend. They may be in a different season than you and have little time to connect with someone else in their lives, but then again, maybe they do. It can't hurt to ask.

Now, if you're generally a person who's gullible, easily swayed, emotionally affected by circumstances around you, or simply influenced easily by others, then you truly need to evaluate your relationships. You may be spending entirely too much time with people who are leading you in a direction that's different from your intended path. If you say, "I don't know what my path is," then that may be the critical idea for you to get first, and then pick relationships carefully. All of us, but especially easily influenced people, need to surround ourselves with people who build us up, encourage us, and give us a good example to follow.

On the other side of the coin is someone who is *not* easily influenced, and, by nature, is a rugged individualist. This person trusts few, admires few, has few if any good friends, and wants to "go it alone." If this is you, then you might want to consider that some of the greatest individuals in the world, regardless of what they accomplished in their lives, had a relationship with a mentor…or two. Some of the finest painters had apprenticeships with masters, but then they went on to become masters themselves; some even more famous than those they learned from.

Look at Luke Skywalker, for example. When he met Yoda, he thought Yoda was amazing and that he could never achieve even a fraction of what the little green dude had. Initially he got frustrated trying to do what he saw Yoda do, trying to be just like Yoda. Later, however, Luke began to grow and become even more skilled than his master by doing things how *he* was designed to do them. And he destroyed the evil empire. Boom.

There are several points to learn here from our *Star Wars* friends. First, Luke felt a connection to Yoda and was somehow drawn to him and what he did. He then spent some time with him to learn what he knew. He had a natural built-in design that led him in that direction and Yoda was willing to teach him. He wasn't "feeling" the work that his uncle had him doing, and he knew that there was something else he was supposed to do. Sound familiar? Many of us know we were called to do something other than what we're doing now.

The point here is to discover the direction that you feel led, and then seek out people who are already on that path. Next, you've got to start doing things that they do, even if it's hard or outside of your current knowledge base or comfort zone. You may get frustrated at first, or even doubt that you can do whatever it is that's in your heart, but you have to continue to work toward it and not give up.

When I set out to write this book, I didn't have any idea what I was doing. If I'd stopped to think about the fact that I wasn't famous, I'd never written a book, and that I didn't have any idea how to get the word out to reach people I thought would benefit from this information, I would've never even started.

Luckily, I surrounded myself with the right relationships. My mentors, wife, family, close friends, and even some of my patients were all relationships that were pivotal to me gaining the confidence I needed to start writing. They were positive, encouraging influences who said to me, "You can do this, and you *need* to do this!" Had I been engulfed in the wrong relationships, I likely would have given up on the dream that God put in my heart.

In the end, surrounding yourself with the right relationships can be the key to unlocking doors that allow you to become who you were designed to be. Who you surround yourself with and how they think and act will often influence your thoughts and actions. If you're caught up in negative relationships, you may never know what life had in store because of your choice to allow the negativity and bad decisions of those people keep you down. Healthy relationships are at the very center of the healthy person you were originally designed to be—they deserve careful focus, effort, and time in order to be successful and helpful.

CHAPTER 7

PLAYTIME

What's the most fun subject to talk about? It's playtime! The fact of the matter is that there are so many different activities that qualify as playtime—it's just that they're different for every person. We were all designed to have specific things that absolutely "float *our* boat," but might mean very little to someone else. That's how you were wired, and it's on purpose. It's not an accident—that's part of your Original Design.

For instance, I really enjoy hunting for ancient arrowheads on ranchland around Texas. When I find one, I like to think about all of the ways humans used to live and it's pretty darn exciting...to me. I have a few on my desk at my office, and most patients will look at them, and say, "What's with the rocks?" I share my excitement and tell how I spent hours in the blazing hot sun, getting filthy dirty and exhausted to find just one. I usually get blank stares and questions like, "Why would you want to do that?"

The cool thing is that many of the other activities that we'll discuss in this book can actually qualify as playtime. For instance, in a few chapters we'll discuss exercise. I know quite a few people who are waiting for the end of the workday with great anticipation so that they can rush to the gym or the trail and "start a-sweatin'."

Many times, playtime is confused with rest because it's often that we do both in the same time period. Let's say you go on vacation to a fabulous destination with crystal clear blue waters, and you decide to float gently in the shallows to look for sea shells with your mask and snorkel. You're smack in the middle of playtime, but at the same time it can be both relaxing and restful.

I do want to make the distinction, however, that playtime isn't always restful and vice versa. If one of your versions of playtime is playing football in the mud, that is awesome but it ain't restful, brother. If you love to close your eyes and lay in the sun, that is restful, but again, it isn't playtime. Part of playtime is that it stimulates a different part of your brain that produces pleasure. It's different than what you might normally do when you're working or at rest.

My wife and I have found that things that seem to be work can become fun if we do them in a certain way. With our kids, it's absolutely true that if we make cleaning up their room a game, and potentially even give them a small prize or treat for completing the "game," they laugh and giggle and have a lot more enthusiasm to get it done. It's because they're now using a different part of their brains. It's interesting what incorporating a little bit of fun can do for our attitude and motivation, whether we're a kid or an adult.

For other people (and these are lucky people by the way), what they do for a living qualifies as playtime because they love what they do so much. It might just be certain aspects of their jobs that they consider as playtime, but it could be that they just have fun in everything they do. This is why my dad has never retired—he *loves* what he does. It's playtime for him!

JEN'S STORY

I'm always telling patients who hate their jobs that they should quit and do something that they love. I had a single patient named Jen who was a customer service agent. She would constantly complain about her boss and tell me how stressed out she was, occasionally in tears. One day I stopped everything and said, "What do you love to do?" She looked a little confused and said, "What do you mean?" I went on to ask her what it was that really got her excited and made her happy. She looked totally confused but finally saw where I was going and said, "Well, I do love dolphins, but it's just something I do for fun. I have no training…I'm not a marine biologist."

I told her not to focus on what she wasn't, but to focus on what she was. She was a girl with a love for dolphins, a passion to help others, and she was bilingual. Long story short, she found a job at a dolphin adventure place in Costa Rica helping English-speaking customers. She met a great guy and got married and is having the time of her life! That's called following your passion and the things that get you all "charged up." You may think it's just playtime. Nope. It's no accident. It's part of your Original Design…and it might just be your purpose.

WE'RE ALL "ADRENALINE JUNKIES"

Our brains need to have all of their areas stimulated or we begin to become someone who is difficult to get along with. In fact, we very well may end up not even liking ourselves. Playtime or having fun and laughing stimulates the part of the brain called the right frontal lobe, and most importantly, the nucleus accumbens, and its connection to the ventral tegmental area (VTA).

Each of us has a unique way that we're wired that gives us a neurochemical "reward" that we experience as pleasure when we're on our designed path.

Research has shown the nucleus accumbens to be the "pleasure center" of the brain. It's the same part of the brain that is stimulated by a good sexual experience, by listening to enjoyable music, or parachuting out of an airplane, if you like that "sorta thang." Some of you would be terrified.

There are multiple parts of the brain that play a role in understanding and appreciating humor, adventure, playing, or just having some "plain ole good, clean fun," so we can't say there's only one part that is the "funny bone" of our brains. In fact, it's our adrenal glands that are in the mid-torso and get their nerve supply from the lower thoracic spine, which produce catecholamines like dopamine, norepinephrine, and epinephrine, or what you may have heard called "adrenaline."

During playtime, a dopamine response is generated from the adrenal glands that stimulates the VTA and nucleus accumbens, which is the natural reward circuitry of our brains. This gives us intense emotions relating to love, excitement, fun, happiness, peace, pleasure, and laughter. This reward circuitry is important. We use it all of the time to try and guide people, our children, or even our pets in the way that we want them to go. When we give a reward, we're reinforcing a behavior that we believe to be beneficial.

Each of us has a unique way that we're wired that gives us a neurochemical "reward" that we experience as pleasure when we're on our designed path. See what I'm saying? Each of us are *designed* to enjoy the things that we do. They're a part of our purpose on earth. That's so cool!

Additionally, the dopamine that your body produces when you're "having fun" can be converted into what are called endorphins and enkephalins. These are our bodies' natural painkillers or "uppers" and act on the body in a similar way to narcotic painkillers like opium, cocaine, heroin, morphine, and methamphetamines. This is why people become "addicted" to doing activities that make them feel good.

Essentially, we're all trying to "feel good." By doing activities that stimulate these areas of our brains, natural "happy chemicals" are made that give us a sense of euphoria or pleasure. Whether our playtime is bungee jumping, enjoying a delicious meal, going on a date, or laughing our booties off at a comedy club, we're all trying to get to the same "happiness destination." Some people's bodies are designed to have certain dopamine receptors that are more stimulated by one activity than another. However, in the end, we're all trying to do the same thing: We all want to feel good! That's the essence of playtime.

**Be fearless in the pursuit of what
"sets your heart on fire," for that's
what you were originally designed to do.**

PLAYTIME HELPS YOU FIND YOUR PURPOSE

It's the discovery of exactly which constructive, beneficial, useful to society (legal) activities that make us feel good that's essentially a personalized defining of what we were originally designed to do. Figuring out and doing *those* things is when people describe feeling "fulfilled." In a word, they're finding their purpose.

We hear so many people say that they just want to do something with their life that's important and makes them feel fulfilled—they want to find their purpose. Clearly, there are many people who get to this point of "fulfillment" but end up in different places. For some, they get "charged" when they're playing a beautiful violin piece in an orchestra performing at Carnegie Hall. For another person, it's caring for and lovingly aiding the elderly; and still for another, it's slam-dunking a basketball right over the head of the defender. Each of them would be extremely unhappy doing the other person's job; it wouldn't be fun (to them) and it's not what they were designed to do.

Every motivational or self-help seminar that I've ever been to tells you that you'll be the most successful at what you're the most passionate about.

Be fearless in the pursuit of what "sets your heart on fire," for that's what you were originally designed to do.

In finding the things that you enjoy and excel at, you're producing a dopamine response and getting excited! This engages the mechanism that God created for you to discover who you were designed to be. How cool is that? Just understanding that what you're excited about is no accident, but is part of your Original Design and purpose on the earth, was worth the cost of this book times a thousand! You're welcome. ☺

Sadly, some people are chasing drugs, alcohol, gambling, indiscriminate sex, overeating of junk foods, or other illegal and immoral behaviors that trigger these same neurochemicals. They're getting a dopamine response, but it's a cheap substitute that will never satisfy and will actually keep them from finding their *true* purpose in life.

We have to protect ourselves from those pitfalls with healthy playtime, healthy eating habits, good friends who give us wise counsel, and a relationship with God and the wisdom that comes with it to help keep us on the right path—the path of our Original Design.

I'M TOO TIRED TO PLAY

One challenge to playtime that I hear from patients all the time is that they're just flat-out pooped! They have no energy to go on a walk, play a game with their kids, read a book, be intimate with their spouse, or go dancing like they used to. Check this out: When we get things out of whack in our overall health, and we prioritize incorrectly and push ourselves to work too hard and get tired, we can experience something called adrenal fatigue.

Remember earlier how I said that the adrenal glands are responsible for producing dopamine and adrenaline and hormones that stimulate all of those receptors in the brain that make us feel good and act as painkillers?

If we're experiencing adrenal fatigue, then we can't get that natural "high." Our pillars of health are out of balance and our foundation of health is beginning to crumble.

We won't enjoy playtime or may not even engage in it at all if we're too tired. Feeling worn out could be from overworking, poor eating habits, depression caused by an unhealthy relationship, disconnection from God, pain in our bodies that's caused by misalignments of the spine or other joints, a lack of sleep, or any other deviation from our Original Design. Along with those problems come the associated side effects of depression, obesity, diabetes, cardiovascular disease, and many others. Are ya startin' to get the idea? Everything works together to either give health or destroy it.

If we aren't making our health a priority, then things are out of balance, and we won't feel good. When we don't feel good, we won't engage in playtime and we won't stimulate the part of the brain that helps us find who we're supposed to be. So we *must* take time for recreation. In fact, if you break down that word, it's "re" and "creation." Playtime helps you to re-create who you were designed to be when you get off track. If we don't play, we'll forget what we're doing in life in the first place, and it can put us in a really bad place. That's no fun and it's dangerous.

Are you starting to see the bigger idea here that connects all of the things we're talking about? It's precisely the understanding of this connection that'll help you see why you're not experiencing the health that you desire. Understanding what's going on can motivate you to make changes that'll put you on the path you were originally designed for. Playtime isn't only a mental vacation that gives you peace and restores balance. It helps you find yourself…your purpose. Make it a priority.

PILLAR II

PHYSICAL

CHAPTER 8

ALIGNMENT

As a chiropractor, I believe that alignment of the spine and all the other joints is absolutely critical to one's overall health. The spine is your body's basic structure, foundation, and framework. Its alignment greatly affects the nerves that run through it and all around it. The structure and function of the entire human body, in fact, is a masterpiece...talk about an amazing Original Design!

So let's start out with some basic anatomy. As an adult, the human body has 206 bones. Between nearly each of these bones, there's a space that's filled with cartilage or connective tissue of some sort that we call a joint. These slippery cartilage-covered joints act as hinges that allow the movement between the bones to be smooth and easy.

The human spine has 24 vertebrae that sit on the sacrum and coccyx, which you'll sometimes hear called the tailbone. Connected to the tailbone is the pelvis or hip bones that house the sockets for the thigh bones. Between each of the vertebra, there's a pad of cartilage called a disc. The disc acts as a spacer plate to allow for nerve roots to come out of the spinal column, and it also acts as a shock absorber (like a thick rubber gasket between two hard objects) to handle the force of gravity and your weight as you walk, jog, jump, or do other physical activities.

IT'S ALL CONNECTED

As you'd imagine, there's an Original Design for the shape of all of these bones and for their connection and relationship to one another. Remember the old song, "♫The hipbone is connected to the thigh bone, the thigh bone is connected to the knee bone…♫"? I sing little bits of it frequently at my office when patients ask me how their foot pain is related to their low back pain.

That reminds me of a patient I had once who came into the office and told me how she sprained her ankle and began to limp. After limping for only a few days, in bad shoes, her knee and hip began to hurt on that same side. After a few more days, she began to have low back pain, then in a few weeks she had upper back pain into her neck, which eventually lead to headaches. And that was the reason she was coming to see me.

When the body's bony framework is taken out of its correct position, (Original Design), weight is distributed inappropriately throughout many of the joints, starting at the feet, and then a domino effect takes place, where one issue creates another issue somewhere else in the chain, and so on. I always tell people not to cheap out on their bed, and don't cheap out on shoes or a good chair for your work station either. You spend a third of your life in bed, but you spend two-thirds of your life on your feet or sitting. Make sure that the majority of the time you're wearing supportive shoes that are comfortable and fit well. Foot damage is the root of many structural problems.

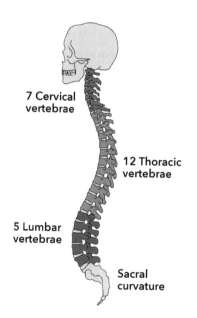

7 Cervical vertebrae

12 Thoracic vertebrae

5 Lumbar vertebrae

Sacral curvature

Anyhow, let's get back to our anatomy lesson. When we look at the spine from the side, it has four curves in it: the cervical curve, the thoracic curve, the lumbar curve, and the sacral curve.

The curves act like shock absorbers or springs that allow your spine to handle force put into it. For example, if you were to jump down off of a box, would you land on your heels with your knees locked, or would you land with a bend at your ankles, knees, and hips? Of course, the answer is bent. The proper curves or arcs are critically important! Your body *knows* that you need to land with a bend in your joints so that you can easily absorb the force that's put into the system. You learned this a long time ago as a little kid.

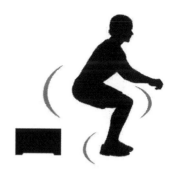

If you landed with your knees locked, then you'd jam all the joints in your lower extremities as well as in your spine. Can you imagine how bad that would hurt? This is why the spine has curves built into it too—to gently absorb force.

THE RAINBOW CURVES

I call those curves the "rainbow curves" because they have a similar degree of curvature to them as a rainbow or the curl of a wave in the ocean, which is an arc or portion of a perfect circle like the cell walls that surround every cell in your body.

Engineers figured out a long time ago that a certain degree of curvature is strong, and they've used it throughout history to build bridges and archways and many other structures that needed strength. Talk about Original Design. How amazing is that?

If we have too much curve *or* too little curve, we have a problem and spinal degeneration begins to occur almost immediately. A study from the Mayo Clinic showed how loss of normal curvature and Forward Head Posture (FHP) causes tension in the TMJ (temporomandibular joint) or jaw, which can lead to pain, headaches, and bite problems.[1]

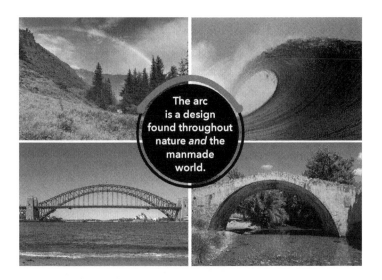

The arc is a design found throughout nature *and* the manmade world.

The study went on to say that uncorrected FHP, over an extended period of time, can cause painful conditions like pinched nerves and blood vessels, altered blood flow to the spinal cord, muscle and tissue pain, fibromyalgia, other soft tissue disorders, and chronic strains. FHP also creates abnormal pressure on the discs that causes them to thin out, make them more prone to be herniated, and create arthritis (bone spurs) all around the edges of the vertebrae.

Many patients will already be aware that they have very little to no normal curve in their necks and significant FHP. When they see their X-rays, it's confirmed.

When you go to a nursing home or retirement community and look at the people who live there, you can't help but notice how many of the folks have a hunched over appearance, sometimes called a "Dowager's hump." This isn't by accident, nor is it a normal part of the aging experience. It may be a common issue that people deal with, but by no means is it designed to occur. It's simply the frequent result of the fact that humans live in a world where the things that we do are in front of and mostly below face level.

Therefore, by definition, we have our head down, and tend to slouch forward to deal with paperwork on a table, read a book, work on a laptop,

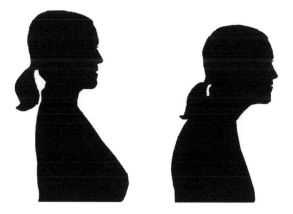

or look at our phones. Take a day to notice all the activities that cause you to bend forward and look down. When you take time to observe this, it's amazing to see just how often this actually occurs. This is a really important issue for our overall health and functionality. It's not a genetic issue. It's not an aging issue. It's not a female or male issue. FHP is a human being issue that we're all susceptible to, but it can be prevented.

Have you ever been doing something else while on the phone, so you hold the phone up to your ear with your shoulder, so you can have your hands free? If you hold it there for an extended period of time, how would it feel when you finally put the phone down and try to straighten out your neck? Ouch!

Nearly all of us have experienced this, so most of us will hold it up to our left ear for a few minutes, switch it to the right ear for a few minutes, and then repeat. The really smart people get a headset or use a speaker phone. Nonetheless, you get my point. In order to keep from hurting yourself, you've figured out over the years that it's important to balance the phone holding equally on the left and the right.

So, let's just apply that same principle of balancing time with the neck bent forward with time backward so we can avoid loss of the "rainbow curve" in our neck from too much FHP. Unless you're Michelangelo and your job is painting the ceiling of the Sistine Chapel in Rome, you're not going to be able to get away from spending time with your head, neck, and upper back being bent forward for far too long. It's what we do *all* day. So guess what we need to do?

We must do exercises that help us keep balance by stretching and strengthening the spine backward to counteract all of the time we spend with our head down and the upper body bent forward. This is critical to create normal posture in the spine, prevent disc and joint damage, and to simply feel good.

Ever notice how when you've been slumping on the couch or at your desk for a while, you begin to hurt, and without even thinking about it, you'll stretch backward and pull your arms back in order to relieve the pain? It feels good, right? That's how well-designed or preprogrammed the body is to maintain balance. You're not even trying to create balance, but by design, you just do it naturally. You inherently know that you need to stretch the other way for a while to even things out.

This reminds me of working with patients who have seizures. Interestingly enough, when we have seizure patients, we often find on X-ray that they have a complete reversal of the normal curvature in the neck. This kind of severe distortion of the Original Design for the neck causes tension on the spinal cord and in certain cases there is a severe spasm or seizure as a result.

What I find interesting is that when the body spasms in a seizure, it violently forces the neck into extension or head backward posture so strongly that it actually causes a little bit of microtearing in the ligaments, tendons, and muscles on the front side of the neck, which then allows the normal cervical curve to come back into the neck enough to take some tension off the spinal cord. The body knows that the reversed curve in the neck is causing major irritation to the cord and exiting spinal nerves and, by design, knows that it needs to force some extension in there to create ease or better function of the whole area.

SCOLIOSIS

When we rotate the picture of the spine so that we're looking at it from the backside, the curves are hidden and it appears to be in a straight line. When there are side-bending or lateral flexion misalignments, it produces curves that shouldn't be there that are collectively called scoliosis. This is commonly when people come to my office and say, "Doc, I'm pretty sure my backbone is all jacked up!" Often, this can easily be seen by family or friends when observing someone in a swimsuit. These misalignments can also cause nerve irritation and joint dysfunction.

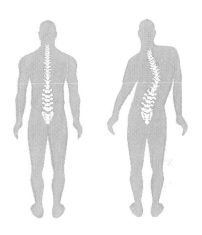

Research has reported that anywhere from 10% to 90% of people have some form of scoliosis. How could it be that varied? It all depends on what you define as scoliosis. Some believe that the curve has to be 40–50 degrees to be considered "real scoliosis," where others believe that even just a few degrees of side-bending or lateral curvature of the spine can technically be considered scoliosis.

Scoliosis screening has been in place in elementary schools for decades. You know the drill. The school nurse will have the kids pull up their shirts and bend forward so they can look at their spines through the skin, from behind. If they see something, they'll send a note home with the child to alert his or her parents to see a doctor. Often, nothing is done, or it's just "watched" until the scoliosis reaches 40 degrees, at which point they may recommend surgery.

Shouldn't we attempt to address the issues before they become that advanced? We may not be able to reverse a severe, aggressively progressing scoliosis, but what if we can slow it down or stop it? I think it's worth a try.

SPINAL ROTATION

The last thing we'll look at in the spine, as far as misalignments are concerned, is rotation. If you put your hand on your back, you can feel the little bumps that are in the middle of the spine, which are called spinous processes. These little bumps should be directly in the center of the spine and in alignment with each other, making a straight line from the base of your skull to your pelvis.

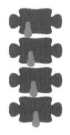 When these little bumps rotate off center, we can get nerve root irritation that also leads to a whole host of problems. Rotation can be extremely painful and cause the "pinch" that people talk about when their back hurts. Whether we're talking about front or back tilting vertebrae, side-bending vertebrae, or rotated vertebrae, these are all painful and damaging alterations of the Original Design for your spine. They significantly affect your overall health but chiropractic can significantly reduce or remove these misalignments.

COMPENSATION

When you look at someone who has a misalignment, you won't see them bent completely over to one side. Rather, you'll see them standing relatively straight, but with perhaps a high shoulder on one side or a high hip, or a twist in any area of the spine due to compensation. The body is designed in such an amazing way that it'll cause other areas of the spine or pelvis to shift out of normal posture to create *overall* stability.

For instance, if the lumbar spine (low back) is leaning to the left due to misalignment, the body will attempt to bend the upper back or neck to the right so that the eyes are level. This is an amazingly good thing. Can you imagine if you tried to drive down the highway at 80 mph with your head bent all the way over to the left? Not a good idea. Your depth perception and spatial relationship recognition would be all out of whack and you'd probably have a wreck and be injured or killed.

It sounds severe, but it's true. The body is often concerned with keeping you comfortable, but it always has self-preservation as the primary objective. If you wreck and die, then nothing else matters, does it? Basically, the body always attempts to keep your feet and your face pointing in the same direction and your eyeballs level with the earth. In order to do this, it has to, technically, put some other things "out of alignment" in order to preserve the overall function and balance of the whole body.

Nature is always creating balance, and so do we. For instance, when you have two heavy grocery bags to carry inside the house, do you put them both in one hand, or one in each hand so that you have equal weight on each side to help you feel balanced? We're always attempting to keep left and right bending, left and right rotation, as well as front bending (flexion) and back bending (extension) in balance…it's a critical part of the Original Design. Like we discussed earlier with FHP, you must create balance to be "at ease" or you will be "dis-eased."

SUBLUXATION

With any of the misalignments that we've discussed, they produce something that's called a subluxation. A *subluxation* is a term that's used to describe a bone that's out of alignment, which then creates a whole list of problems. Just a few of those problems are improper motion in the joint, nerve irritation, pain, muscle spasm, inflammation, arthritis, degeneration, weakness, and dysfunction in many different ways.

When joints are subluxated, they may still partially function but not to the extent that they're designed to. Think of a sliding glass door that's out of its track. You may still be able to slide it, but it's going to be difficult and it'll grind and make noise. If these subluxations are left uncorrected, they can significantly affect your normal every day life or even your ability to do your job. It could be anywhere from something simple like brushing hair all the way to the extreme of not even being able to move without pain. Normal function and life can just…stop.

When I began to work on Andy Roddick in 2004, he was the number one tennis player in the world. He was having siginificant pain and decreased range of motion in the neck, upper back, shoulder and down the arm to the hand. He had weakness in that arm that resulted in the inability to hold the racquet tightly which caused decreased serve strength. After an exam and x-rays, we identified subluxations in his spine, shoulder, elbow and wrist and began to adjust him. That December, at the Davis Cup, the pain and stiffness were gone, the strength was back and he broke the world record for serve speed at 155 mph. #ChiropracticWorks

You can have a subluxation in any joint in the body from the spine to the fingers, wrists, elbows, shoulders, toes, ankles, knees, and hips. Pretty much any joint in the body that has motion in it can be subluxated. This is what chiropractors deal with every day in their offices.

When a vertebra gets subluxated, it can irritate one or more of the spinal nerves that exit the spine, and a person can begin to experience many if not all of the issues I discussed above. Often the first thing they feel is pain. Within a short period of time, muscle spasms begin as a reaction of the body which acts as a self-protective mechanism to keep that area from moving. Like a brace, spasms keep you from creating greater irritation. Then inflammation or swelling sets in as the body is further protecting and repairing the damaged area.

Wanna guess what three of the most commonly used medications in the world are? You guessed it! Painkillers, muscle relaxers, and anti-inflammatories—the three medications that seek to alleviate the symptoms of subluxations. As we all know, you can take one or all of these medications and maybe get some temporary relief from the symptoms, but they'll never change the *underlying* condition that's creating your symptoms. It's like smashing the smoke alarm instead of putting out the fire! It doesn't make a lot of sense.

Often, underlying issues are undetectable and don't create pain until pressure is put on them. It's like not knowing you have a rock in your shoe until you actually stand on it and begin walking. What chiropractic seeks to do is to find the source of the issue and remove it so that the body can heal itself.

Again, not only can people experience those last three symptoms, but they can also begin to have some other functional issues within the body, like Andy did. Just ask anyone who's walked out of a chiropractor's office after being carried in only minutes before, while in severe pain. But it doesn't just have to be muscular dysfunction. It can be many different functional issues…even some unusual ones.

JUDY'S STORY

That reminds me of a patient named Judy. She had an amazing experience with an adjustment for something that I'd never seen before. Here's her story in her own words:

> While remodeling a home and living in the dust, I woke one night with a horrible headache. I went into the bathroom for some aspirin only to see in the mirror extreme swelling from below my chin to the top of my scalp. My ear stood straight out and my eye was almost shut! I kind of looked like the "elephant man." My ear and face were burning hot.

> We went straight to the ER and proceeded to stun every nurse and doctor who walked into my room. I was scheduled to fly out of town soon, but was told that was not possible, as I had cellulitis which was too close to my brain. Any extra pressure could cause a big problem with further infection. After three days of traditional

treatment, daily IVs, multiple antibiotic shots, and pills, there was *no change.*

The next day, while sitting with my husband during his chiropractic adjustment, Dr. Mark asked questions about my condition. He suggested an adjustment for me. I agreed as I was very frustrated with the lack of any improvement. He adjusted my whole spine, including my neck, which was extremely sore.

We were on our way home when there was a moment I'll never forget. It hadn't been more than *20 minutes after* the adjustment that I felt a sensation of cool water running from behind my ear down my neck. I even touched it…it was that real, but nothing was there. By evening, there was a distinct reduction in the swelling and redness of my face, and by the morning it was gone.

Two days later, I was off on my flight to California. The head and neck specialist said it was the meds "finally kicking in," but I know exactly what happened. Thanks, Dr. Mark, for helping my body heal itself!

That's such a cool story, but it's not what normally brings people in to see us. As you'd imagine, when people come to see a chiropractor, they don't often come in and say, "Hey, Doc, I think I have a little nerve irritation in my neck that's creating pressure on the nerves to the glands in my neck, and I believe they might be dysfunctioning and swelling." No, they come in and say, "My neck hurts."

So, of course, our first goal is to always remove the nerve irritation to relieve their pain. But we're also interested in ensuring that any organs or muscles that are connected to the subluxated areas are getting optimal nerve supply and therefore functioning as well as they can.

DYSFUNCTION: THE REST OF THE STORY

Many people understand the concept of a pinched nerve, but usually they're only thinking about the pain associated with it. The pain they're feeling is associated with the sensory part of the nerve function which creates sensations like heat, burning, cold, itching, tingling, and tickling. There's another side to the story, though.

As we discussed in Judy's story, dysfunction is another result of subluxation. The nerve roots that exit the spine don't just control pain but also play a role in the function of organs, muscles, and other tissues that receive some kind of nerve supply from that same region. Think of nerve compression like a dimmer switch to a light. If you turn down the flow of electricity to the light, it may still work but not to its full potential. Subluxations can do the same thing to our bodily functions.

For instance, in the lumbar spine, nerves that exit the spine don't just give you sensations in the low back, but they also play a role in the function of your bowel, bladder, and sphincter muscles, as well as reproductive and other organs. If an orthopedic surgeon suspects that you may have a disc herniation that's creating pressure on the nerve roots in the low back, they may ask you as part of their normal exam if you've experienced any changes in your bowel or bladder habits. That may sound like a strange question, but there's a really good reason for asking it.

They know that if you've been losing control of either one, a disc herniation may be causing nerve root compression in the lumbar spine. The pain is caused by the irritation to the sensory function of the nerve and the organ dysfunction is caused by irritation to the motor function of the nerve. This reminds me of a young man who came to my office with only a little pain in the low back, but a great deal of dysfunction due to his subluxations. Here's his story.

JAXSON'S STORY

Jaxson came into my office a few weeks before his sixteenth birthday with bowel incontinence that he'd endured since he was eight years old. He had accidents one to three times per day, each day of those eight years, and was really burning through underwear due to the leakage. The smell was definitely noticeable, and you can imagine what other kids at school were saying. It was emotionally exhausting, yet he had a really good attitude about it. I was so impressed with him.

His parents were extremely proactive and over the years, had tried everything, including multiple medications, enemas, acupuncture, special diets, and a program called brain balance. None of it helped. They were at the end of their rope. So after seeking an orthopedic surgeon's opinion and an MRI, surgery was performed on his lumbar spine when he was 14. Still, *nothing changed*. They were all disappointed and were beginning to lose hope.

As a last resort, his mom brought him to our office. After locating spinal and pelvic misalignments on an X-ray, we began adjusting him. His parents and grandparents were faithful to bring him in regularly to get adjusted, and it paid off. He began to see immediate improvement. Where he'd been averaging roughly 60 "accidents" per month, after his third month of care, he had only two! Not only could he now feel it when the urge came, but he was able to hold it and get to the restroom in time.

Here are Jaxson's own words: "This totally changed my life and it was working the second week of going. I'm just about clean all day, every day… my life has been so much better!" That's life-changing stuff right there. He and I and his family were all extremely happy with the results! When the spine is restored to its Original Design, good things happen.

Motion is the key to joint health.

OSTEOARTHRITIS: IT'S NOT JUST FOR OLD PEOPLE

There's one more major factor about subluxation that we're concerned with, called degeneration or degenerative joint disease (DJD), which causes bone spurs, also commonly referred to as osteoarthritis. It's a direct result of bones being out of position and "rubbing" too hard on the disc or cartilage in between. Initially, there's only the subluxation and the vertebra is kind of "stuck" out of place and doesn't move normally. Over time, it begins to diminish the flow of fluids in and out of the disc area. The *only* way that the joint stays properly hydrated is by motion. Motion is the key to joint health.

This is called joint imbibition, which means the disc is imbibing or drinking in the fluid surrounding the joint. Without proper motion, the disc becomes dehydrated like a prune and eventually shrivels up. It becomes thinner and can't perform its two jobs: being a shock absorber and being a spacer plate to leave room for the nerve to come out. This isn't just for older people; it can happen at nearly any age.

When the bones of the spine have been out of alignment for many years, the discs aren't of much use. Eventually the disc or cartilage is so thinned out and dried up that the bones begin to rub on each other. Arthritis begins and the bone spurs start to grow together, creating a fusion where there's little to no motion left. It's limiting and can be quite painful in the process.

One of the goals of chiropractic is to prevent or at least slow down the progression of osteoarthritis. By keeping the joints in alignment and moving normally, the fluids surrounding the discs, or any joint for that matter, can keep the joint lubricated and healthy. Motion is lotion.

MANY THINGS RESPOND TO CHIROPRACTIC

There are countless stories from around the world of people who've been in pain, muscle spasms, or inflammation, and unable to function normally, if at all. After having adjustments to the affected body parts, they report having seemingly "miraculous" recoveries, restoration of normal function, and pain relief. They weren't miracles, just the simple restoration of health by aligning the spine and other joints to the Original Design.

On a daily basis in my office we hear these words: "That feels so much better, Doc. Thank you!" The basic premise of chiropractic is simple: When your spine and the other joints of your body are in alignment, you'll feel great and function well. If they aren't…you won't.

SARAH'S STORY

I remember one patient in my first few months of practice who was about 20 years old, athletic, and full of life. She'd been in a head-on car accident without airbag deployment. While the impact was only at about 20 mph, the other person was traveling at about 20 mph as well, which meant that the actual impact to her body was about 40 mph. As you might imagine, she had injuries from head to toe.

First and foremost, she had pain throughout the spine, which is commonly called whiplash. We worked on her neck, upper back, low back, pelvis, sacrum, shoulders, collarbone, sternum, and front ribs where she was bruised from the seatbelt. She began to improve nicely in every area over the course of eight weeks or so, when one day she pushed herself off of the table in an unusual way and she screamed in pain. I, of course, asked her what was wrong and she stated that she'd been dealing with thumb and wrist pain ever since the accident.

I asked her why she didn't tell me about it before, to which she answered, "I didn't think you worked on wrists." I felt like I failed for not having told her that we work on *every* joint in the body…every single day. They should really call chiropractors joint doctors instead of back doctors, as we work on any joint in the body that moves.

Anyway, she stuck out her thumb and wrist and said, "Please tell me there's something you can do for this—I've tried everything." She went on to explain that since the accident, with all the pain she'd been having in the thumb and wrist area, she'd been to three different doctors, had three shots of cortisone, anti-inflammatories, painkillers, muscle relaxers, wrist bracing, and an MRI. Next, they were going to try exploratory surgery to see "what the heck was keeping this thing from healing." Since her insurance had run out of coverage, she had to pay for the MRI out of pocket, to the tune of $1,000.

I looked at her thumb and wrist, did some standard orthopedic and neurological tests, and then adjusted it as I had thousands of other wrists and thumbs before hers. There was a loud "pop" (which doesn't always happen, or need to happen, to be effective) and she let out a little, "Ouch." Then she said, as she was moving it around, "Hey, that feels way better!" After two more adjustments, she never complained of her wrist and thumb again. That was it! Are you kidding me?

This always leads me to wonder what is going on in our health-care system when so many health-care professionals examined her for the same condition and no one addressed the actual problem, which was just a simple "jammed" thumb? She'd been gripping the steering wheel so tightly during the accident that when the impact happened, it caused a significant compression of the wrist and thumb joint complex, as well as all of her spinal misalignments.

Why did she have to go eight weeks with life-altering pain and dysfunction, spend thousands of dollars, subject her body to multiple toxic medications, and hours of treatment, only to have the problem fixed by *pulling her finger*? (No laughing.) Seriously, though. What's wrong with this picture?

Shouldn't we have a simple, methodical, conservative approach to health care that only increases in cost, risk to the patient, and complexity of care if the patient isn't improving? In other words, if you don't get better with natural, noninvasive, gentle treatments that have little to no risk, like chiropractic care, nutritional counseling, physical therapy, and massage, *then* you should take more dangerous and invasive steps. Oh well, maybe someday.

WHEN SHOULD I SEE A CHIROPRACTOR?

I would suggest that you need to have a chiropractor do a basic alignment check as a part of the initial evaluation of most nonemergency conditions. Clearly, if there's a fracture, a cancer, or some other disease process that has gone way too far, that person needs emergency medical care as soon as possible. Honestly, if I fall off a cliff, I don't want some vitamins and a massage; I want heavy narcotics and the best ER surgeons available.

I simply question, as I believe all patients should, the appropriateness of any treatment. If you have a sore back or a headache, let's not have surgery be our first option, but our last. There are many conservative options for treating nearly anything in a natural, noninvasive way that can and should be tried first. When they're needed, the advances of modern medicine are incredible and can save lives. There's always a time and place for that kind of care.

As far as chiropractic care is concerned, you should see a chiropractor for practically any musculoskeletal and joint issue. We see patients for headaches, neck, back, pelvic, hip, knee, ankle, foot, toe, shoulder, elbow, wrist, hand, and finger pain. Pretty much anytime your body's structure or frame gets misaligned, it can cause dysfunction and hurt. When you notice that something is continually bothering you and it won't go away, it's a good time to see a chiropractor!

Little misalignments create a little pain and dysfunction, large misalignments create significant pain and dysfunction, and major dislocations can cause severe pain and paralysis, or even death. The further we get away from the Original Design for our spines, like any area of health, the bigger the problems become. It's like a car, a bicycle, or anything else with a frame: If it's bent out of shape, it doesn't work correctly. If your low back is misaligned, it throws off the alignment of the pelvis, the hip, the knee, the ankle, and the foot, and now the whole chain is "jacked up."

AUDREY'S STORY

That reminds me of another story of a little girl whose mom brought her fifteen-month-old toddler in...who *wasn't* toddling. She would only crawl, and with only one leg! She'd been trying to walk for months but would crumble under the one leg that wasn't working right.

They had tried everything to help get her walking, but nothing medical was helping. Her pediatrician finally told them "Don't worry about it until she's two years old." They came to our office, we checked her out, and I did a few simple, gentle adjustments. She smiled the whole time. They took her home and set her down in the middle of the living room floor, where there wasn't even anything to hold on to in order to pull herself up. They took a video of what happened next.

Here's her excited mommy's story: "Our little girl just stood up and took her first few steps the very same day as her *first* adjustment! She had never been able to take steps or stand up by herself like she does in the video and she's 15 months old! I'm so glad chiropractic help was suggested for her!" (Check out her video on my website.)

BUILD A TEAM OF MEDICAL PROFESSIONALS

Every person should have a team of health-care providers from different specialties whom they trust. You must know your doctors, nurses, and therapists, and have similar beliefs and goals as they pertain to your overall health. You might have a doctor who thinks nutrition, exercise, prayer, and chiropractic is a waste of time, but *you* consider them to be integral parts of what you do to keep yourself healthy. You're not likely to have positive interactions with or feel good about that doctor, and therefore not receive the kind of care you need and deserve. If this were the case, I would suggest that it'd be time to find a different doctor.

You want a team of people who are willing to work with others on the team and who are willing to listen to you and your concerns. This is not to say that you shouldn't listen to the wisdom and experience of trained medical professionals, but rather that the decisions made regarding your health should be agreed upon by all, especially by you.

I, of course, believe that your team should have a good chiropractor on it who can analyze your frame and determine if it's in the alignment that it was originally designed to be in. All the amazing stories of the "chiropractic miracles" that you've read weren't miracles at all. They were just people with spinal misalignments that happened to have some awesome side effects after being adjusted. Chiropractic is safe, gentle and effective. You've got nothing to lose by getting checked. What are you waiting for? Millions of people can't be wrong…so just ask a friend who they see. Give your body the best chance it can have at optimal health and keep it aligned to its Original Design!

CHAPTER 9

EXERCISE

All right, I know, I know. Most of you hate exercise. I heard one comedian say, "I'd probably do more exercise, but it's just that the weights are so heavy!" Seriously though, when you think about it, haven't there been times in your life where you've been sweatin' like a pig, burnin' calories like crazy, and you didn't even realize that you were exercising?

That's it! Having *fun* is the secret to great exercise that will make it easy for you keep it a consistent habit in your life. It has a lot to do with your state of mind.

When my kids are hiking a trail with my wife and me, they sometimes start whining and complaining that their legs are tired and that they're thirsty. Can you hear them? "I'm tired! It's hot!" However, as soon as they see the waterfall in the distance, or they spontaneously begin a game of tag, the fun takes over, and all of a sudden they're full of energy and bouncing down the trail. It's not the body that is often the real problem with getting exercise, but the attitude.

WHAT SHOULD I DO AND WHEN SHOULD I DO IT?

Do whatever you want for exercise, but do *something*, and do it often. I'll typically tell patients to exercise first thing in the morning if possible. This gets your body going and you get your metabolism kicked into gear. But some people just aren't "early birds." The second best would be to exercise no later than lunchtime; it'll get you charged for the second half of your day. I don't recommend exercising in the late evening, because that can really throw off your body's rhythm and affect your sleep. But if you have no other time to do it, it might work for you.

I'll say it again. What you do for exercise needs to be something that you enjoy…at least a little bit. When you're having fun, it doesn't matter what you're doing because you won't think about exercise as a chore anymore. It could be a sport you love to play, slow-burn exercises, lifting weights, jogging, mall walking, Pilates, Yoga, aerobics, Jazzercise, dance, martial arts, trampoline, or participating in the "running of the bulls" in Spain. (That last one's a little dangerous.) ☺

Seriously, whatever works! You could even put on some music that you love and start "♪gettin' jiggy wid it.♫" (For those of you over 55, that means dancing.) Moving around, getting your blood pumping, and using your muscles is the important thing here, not what you're doing.

Something I try to hammer home with all my patients is that motion is the key to joint health. My friend Charles memorized that phrase and can quote it to me on demand. He's made changes in his daily life regarding exercise and getting up from his desk every so often to stretch that have benefited him in many ways. We can all benefit from simply moving more— it barely takes any time from our day, but the benefits are tremendous. Look at your day and think of times where you're sedentary for far too long. Then try to come up with creative ways to get moving. Remember the old adage, "Move it or lose it." It's so true for all of us.

Nearly everything in life requires maintenance. If you think you're going to be healthy without maintaining your body, then you're going to be disappointed as time goes on. We can't expect optimal health unless we take care of what we have. The body was designed in such a way that if it doesn't get movement, its muscles begin to atrophy or shrink and wither away. Obviously, this means that we become weaker and less able to move around and do the things that we'd like to do, so we have to come up with ways to counter this.

I strategize with patients all the time about ways to get movement or stretching or exercise in during their normal day while not even taking away time from what they want to do. For instance, I often suggest to patients who are going to watch an hour or so of TV that they simply stand up and move around or stretch, or do ab crunches or push-ups during the commercial breaks. The average commercial breaks add up to about 15 minutes per hour of TV. Think about that. You can get in a 30-minute workout while watching two hours of TV!

Now while I'd never advocate watching two hours of TV every day, you get the idea. You can make use of the time that you have if you just stop to think about it, make a plan, and then simply start doing it. Do some simple exercises by bending forward, backward, side to side, and swiveling the hips in circles in both directions (which I call the Elvis pelvis).

What you do in life is bigger than you.

If you drive for a living, or you're simply running a few errands, you can do abdominal exercises while sitting in the car. Whether at work or at home, if you've been at your desk for too long, then simply get up and do sixty seconds of stretching, go get a drink of water, go to the bathroom, or simply walk the hallways for a little bit. The key is to never stay in one position for too long. We were designed to move. So let's get off our gluteus maximuses (some gluteuses are more "maximus" than others) and get moving!

For those of you who love exercise—I *do* love you—but you must know that you are weird. Don't be sad that many people despise you—they're just jealous that they don't love to work out too. If you can't wait to get back to the gym, or in the pool, or on the track, this piece of the puzzle will be easy for you. However, it's still good for you and all of us to learn *why* exercise is so valuable. I promise that you'll learn something, and I might even encourage you to inspire someone you love to begin an exercise program that could help save his or her life. It's amazing how what we do in our lives becomes an example for our families, our friends, our coworkers, and everyone in our circles of influence.

Being healthy is contagious. Making a decision right now to start exercising, could inspire someone else to do the same and may save a life. What you do in life is bigger than you. That's part of the Original Design too. We're supposed to focus on others more than ourselves.

WHAT GOOD IS EXERCISE ANYWAY?

Let's discuss the benefits of exercise. Exercise affects so many other areas of health and life. The benefits are surprisingly far-reaching and it's important for each of these areas to function in the way that they were originally designed. It all works together for a reason.

The first talk that I ever gave, "The Seven Habits of Highly Healthy People," had a section devoted to the many benefits of exercise. As I was doing the research for it, I was blown away by the number of interconnected benefits. When looking up how sleep was affected by exercise, I'd find a study that also linked it to improving emotional health. When exploring how exercise helps muscles, I'd stumble across research that showed how it was valuable for losing weight or lowering blood pressure too. In the end, exercise was a common thread that was reported to benefit every other area of health.

One study, published in the Archives of Internal Medicine in 1999, divided 156 men and women with depression into three separate groups. One group took part in an aerobic exercise program, another took antidepressants, and the third group did both.

After 16 weeks, depression had lessened in all three groups. About 60%–70% of the people in all three groups could no longer be classified as having major depression! These findings suggest that for those who want or need to avoid drugs, exercise might be an acceptable substitute for antidepressants. A follow-up to that study found that the effects of exercise lasted longer than those of antidepressants.

Researchers followed up with 133 of the original patients six months after the first study ended.[1] They found that the people who exercised regularly after completing the study, regardless of which treatment they were on during the study, were less likely to relapse into depression.

As I mentioned in the Introduction, all four pillars of health are affected by regular exercise. The benefits of exercise are all clearly intertwined and support one another. Here are a few of them that most of us would love to have:

- Energy: When you exercise, you'll get tons of energy that you've never had before.

- Strength: You'll get the strength to help you do everything you need to do, from wrestling with the kids to Zebra wrestling (which is very common in Zimbabwe). ☺

- Sleep: Studies show that you'll get more sleep, fall asleep more easily, stay asleep better, and wake up more refreshed because you'll get more *restful* sleep after exercising.

- Antidepressant effect: Research shows that exercise works as well as antidepressant medications for depression and lasts longer than the meds too.

- Pain relief: You'll also be producing endorphins, enkephalins, and dynorphins, which are the body's natural painkillers.

- Joint health: The motion of exercise also lubricates the joints. Remember? Motion is lotion!

- Self-esteem: You'll feel better about yourself because you'll like what you see in the mirror. You'll also produce other neurotransmitters in the brain that give a greater sense of well-being.

- Fitness modeling jobs: Did I mention you'd get the ripped abs you've always wanted? I'm kidding, but it's true (with a proper diet).

- Injury prevention: As the muscle fibers develop and your muscles get stronger, you'll have stronger ligaments and tendons too, which helps prevent injury.

- Blood pressure: Multiple studies show how exercise can significantly reduce blood pressure and give your blood vessels a much-needed rest from all the pounding.

- Stress: People who exercise regularly report significantly lower levels of stress and are less likely to have a nervous breakdown or any form of anxiety.

- Stability: Through increased muscle tone and connective tissue strength, your spine and all the joints in your body will be more durable and less likely to get misaligned.

- Cleansing: You'll cleanse your body by sweating as the skin empties toxins from all your systems when you start drippin' with sweat. (I realize that women glisten and men sweat—my wife made me aware of this.)

- Weight control: When it comes to losing weight, exercise not only helps you to burn calories when you're actually exercising, but it helps to change your metabolism too.

This means that as you exercise, you'll begin to burn calories when you're at rest more than if you didn't exercise. You can also lose weight much faster and safer when you're exercising.

- Mental clarity: Exercise should and needs to be a part of your weekly schedule. It helps to keep your mind sharp and focused. Make time for it—you'll be glad you did.

- Spiritual health: Exercise honors God with your body and provides the opportunity to see how the design of the body is truly a masterful creation. It prompts us to be thankful for how amazingly well it works. What a gift it is!

ARE SOME EXERCISES BETTER THAN OTHERS?

Patients will often ask me about the "best" exercises. As I stated earlier, the best exercise really is the one that you'll actually do on a regular basis. The best exercise in the world is of absolutely no value to you if you don't do it. When I think of ideal exercises, though, I think of how I see exercises affect my patients.

High-impact exercises like boxing, kickboxing, marathon running, football, or otherwise anything that really jars your body *can* create as much or more harm than overall good for your body. That being said, don't let me stop you from doing the things you love, just consider mixing those in with exercises that are less damaging to the body. This is called cross-training. As we age, this becomes extremely important for maintaining good functional long-term health that allows us to live the life we want to.

I often encourage heavy weight lifters to consider lightening the weight and increasing repetitions a little over time as they get older. Likewise, I encourage aging runners to consider adding some lower impact exercise to diminish the damage done by "pounding the pavement." High-impact exercises can beat you up. It's a simple matter of wear and tear. Anything that's used frequently, with heavy force applied to it, will wear out quicker than something that's treated a bit more gently.

Imagine finding a 1957 Chevy two-door with those heavy doors made of solid steel. Let's suppose that it was owned by a single guy who just couldn't get a date, and only had the passenger door opened and closed once a week when he took his mother to church. However, he slams *his* door shut multiple times per day, every day since 1957. Now over 60 years later, on which side of the car do you think the door hinges are still working smoothly and properly, and which side has worn-out, beat-up hinges? It's just a simple by-product of heavy use and abuse.

I'm absolutely *not* saying that we shouldn't use our joints, but only that we should be wise in choosing exercises that limit damage and focus more on smooth motions to create strength. This will help ensure that our joints work extremely well as we get into our 70s, 80s, and 90s. They're absolutely designed to work that long or longer if we take good care of them.

The athletes with the *best* bodies are ones whose core muscles (lower back, lower abdominals, and side-stabilizing muscles like the quadratus lumborum, iliopsoas, and obliques) are extremely strong. They tend to work their entire body and are in good cardiovascular condition too. A good example of this would be swimmers. They have great symmetry from side to side due to using both arms and both legs equally. Some athletes like golfers who swing one direction all the time, or baseball players who throw with one arm, tend to get stronger muscles on one side, which is not ideal.

The best exercises also create good muscle symmetry from front to back. Some male weight lifters might be tempted to work on the front side or "chick-magnet muscles" like the biceps, pecs, and abs while ignoring their back and side muscles.

Last, ideal exercise works both the top and the bottom. Where a power hitter in baseball might have a really powerful chest, shoulders, and arm muscles, they might have a flabby stomach and weaker legs by comparison. (No offense to Babe Ruth—he was the best!)

I personally love to hike because it's less impact than jogging, and I get to be outside where I can connect with nature, pray, think, and get a serious leg and core workout. However, it doesn't provide much upper body challenge, so I add in upper body exercises by lifting weights on the days that I'm not hiking. Again, I recommend doing what works best for you.

However, if I were forced to give a short list of *conventional* exercises that are the most beneficial while being lower impact and gentle on the body, then, in no particular order, I'd say:

1. Swimming (or water aerobics for the elderly)

2. Rowing or ski machine with an arm attachment

3. Full-body circuit training with weights

4. Bicycling, hiking, or fast walking (plus some additional upper body work)

5. Elliptical or Gazelle type gliding machine with an arm attachment

6. Pilates, Yoga or Tai Chi

7. Unicycling while juggling five-pound weights

I'm kidding about number seven, if you hadn't figured that out yet. Doing that for exercise might cause you to end up in the hospital. This would not help in achieving your Original Design for health. ☺

Ideally, I'd recommend getting exercise six days per week. They don't all have to be intense workouts, but they need to get the heart rate up, the blood pumping, and the muscles and joints moving. I also strongly believe in taking one day off per week to let everything rest, including your mind, body, and spirit. If God rested on the seventh day, then I figure it's probably a good idea for us too! Don't you think?

The ranges of motion that you consistently use are the ones that you keep.

STREEEEEEETCHING

Now let's talk about stretching for just a little bit. When we talk about flexibility, the only way to keep something flexible is to continue to stretch it and require it to bend on a regular basis. If your body doesn't move regularly, it loses the range of motion that you were designed to have. To get technical, the ligaments that hold joints together experience something called "creep" when they're not being used. This means that they shorten and pull the joints closer together, which restricts the range of motion. To put it plainly, you get tight, or as they say in the country, "you get all stove up."

I've had patients get frozen shoulder syndrome simply from never moving their arms more than to type at a keyboard or to stick a sandwich in their "pie hole." The ranges of motion that you consistently use are the ones that you keep. If there happens to be one you don't want anymore, just stop doing it! Just kidding. Don't do that. Not all of us are destined to be in Cirque du Soleil, though, so don't be upset if you can't rest your head on your tailbone when bending backward. Some people are definitely wound tighter than others, so just stretch to what *feels* comfortable for you. You'll get more range of motion over time, the longer you stretch.

It's way more important to get some motion on a frequent basis than to be able to put your palms on the floor when bending forward at the hips. Extreme stretching isn't necessary and doesn't benefit the joints as much as regular motion in many different directions.

Most of us want to be "active" in our old age and be able to travel and play with the grandkids. We have to think about the kind of lifestyle we want down the road and start making choices now that will get us to our goals. The surest way I know how to do that for muscle and joint function is to simply "♫Keep on movin', don't stop, no!♫" (Remember that song from the 80's?) My girls said that Dory would say, "Just keep swimming."

So, listen, stretches are fairly simple: Move any given joint through all of the directions that it can move, and do it regularly. You can do anything from simple floor stretches to other methods like Yoga, Pilates, Tai Chi. You can get exercise-specific muscle group stretches for runners, tennis players, golfers, etc. from your chiropractor, physical therapist, or personal trainer.

As I conclude this chapter on exercise, there's a scripture that fits very well here, as it helps us put our health in the right perspective. My wife even wrote it on the mirror in our workout room at home. It reads: "Do you not know that your bodies are temples of the Holy Spirit, who is in you, whom you have received from God? You are not your own; you were bought at a price. Therefore honor God with your bodies" (1 Corinthians 6:19–20). It always reminds me how to treat my body and why it's so important to exercise, stretch, eat right, and generally take care of and maintain the Original Design of the amazing bodies that we've been given.

CHAPTER 10

REST

Rest can generally be categorized as any activity where your body and mind, and hopefully your spirit, are at ease. Sleep is what most people think of when they hear the word *rest*, but other things can be restful too. For example, taking a nap, relaxing, going to church, going on a vacation, lying on the beach, snuggling, listening to peaceful music, prayer, meditation, taking a hot bath, reading a calming book, sitting under a shade tree on a hot summer day, and a good night's sleep can all be forms of rest.

When you've been going full speed ahead and wearing yourself out, you've got to employ one technique or another of rest. In fact, your body will function best with some rest between periods of activity. For me, it's extremely restful when I can get away from all the cares of the world with a hike in the mountains where I can smell the pine trees and hear an eagle call out, or a trip to the beach where I can stick my toes in the sand and breathe fresh ocean air. Connecting with nature is something that we were designed to do. When we experience the beauty and vastness of what God created in the great outdoors, it's totally re-energizing.

A really interesting book called *Earthing* explores the rejuvenating effect of connecting with the earth. Some of the science could be questioned, but the undeniable truth is that we, as humans, feel better when we disconnect from the man-made "concrete jungle" and connect with the natural world.

However, even a short break to stretch or a walk to the water cooler can be restful. It can clear your mind and help you tackle the rest of your afternoon work. You'll stay awake better and find that you have improved focus. Above all, though, you need sleep.

**Your body will function best with
some rest between periods of activity.**

YOU'RE FEELING VERY SLEEPY...

A typical night's sleep is divided into five or more cycles that repeat throughout the night. Each cycle is made up of different stages that all have unique characteristics:[1]

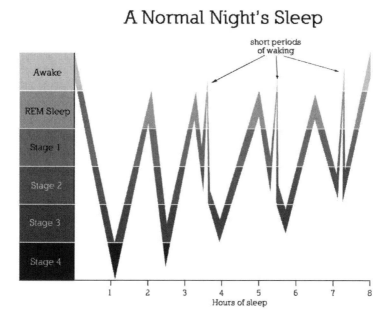

A Normal Night's Sleep

- Stage 1: This is light sleep as you're initially drifting off. It lasts 5–10 minutes and you can be easily awakened during this time.

- Stage 2: This is slightly deeper but still considered light sleep. Your brain waves change, and it lasts 10–25 minutes.

- Stage 3: Delta (brain wave) sleep begins and heart rate and blood pressure begin to slow. This stage lasts only a few minutes.

- Stage 4: Lasting 20–40 minutes, this is our deepest sleep and it's the hardest to wake from. Brain and nerve activity slows, and a growth hormone for body repair is released.

- REM sleep: This type of sleep is when we dream and the body consolidates memories. Our skeletal muscles are effectively paralyzed during this stage. Each successive cycle is longer through the night, up to about an hour.

Each stage is important, but rapid eye movement or REM sleep seems to be especially critical to our health. Research from the American Sleep Association shows that rats, which normally live for three years, will only live *five weeks* without REM sleep and three weeks with no sleep at all.

The body must "power down" in order to repair all of the damage that was done from the previous day's activities. The deepest and most restorative sleep occurs in stage 4, between 10 p.m. and 2 a.m. After that, sleep becomes more superficial and it's harder to fall back asleep.[2]

Sleep is the time of the day that we do the bulk of repair and regeneration in our bodies. Think of it this way: If you owned a restaurant and you had a busy day, you'd have to clean up all the mess that was made from that day's business, and then you'd have to prep for the following day by getting food ready before the customers showed up. In the same way, our bodies need to have time to get ready for the next day by recharging and repairing all of our systems. If we go and go and take no time to rest, then our bodies can't function normally.

If we frequently get inadequate sleep, our bodies will run out of fuel and resources to conduct normal activities. Immunity will be reduced, thereby increasing our risk of getting sick. Hormone levels will be disrupted or depleted, which can cause us to be unusually angry, sensitive, or simply unable to cope with regular situations that wouldn't normally be a problem at all. Our energy levels will be severely affected and we'll feel like we're just dragging all the time, and don't seem to have the energy to do even simple activities. This is not how we were originally designed to live. We need to get in a good rhythm.

As the sun sets and darkness takes over, our bodies begin to produce melatonin, which is a chemical that naturally makes us sleepy.[3] When the sun comes up and light increases, we wake up. That's the Original Design for our sleep which sets our internal clock, aka our circadian rhythm. When we start to get sleepy at the same time every night, and wake up one minute before our alarm clock goes off, then we're in a good rhythm.

TIPS FOR GOOD SLEEP

My wife and I have figured out (and have to keep telling ourselves) that if we don't get enough rest, we're simply not going to be healthy. We've found that a good night of sleep is an absolute key for staying healthy. Not that it's rocket science, but we've even noticed that when our kids miss even a few hours of sleep, they're cranky, don't think clearly, are much more quick to cry, and simply can't seem to cope with life as well.

I know beyond a shadow of a doubt that every time I've been sick in the last 15 years, lack of sleep was always a huge factor. Without proper sleep, research shows that your immune system and overall health will suffer.[4] Here are some tips that can help you get better sleep:

- Get exercise during the day, preferably in the morning. This creates a natural sleepy effect at the end of the day that helps you go to and stay asleep.

- Get a good, comfortable, and supportive mattress. You spend a third or your life in bed. It's worth spending money on something this important.

- Don't drink anything about two hours before bedtime if you have issues waking up to urinate. The kidneys need about 90 minutes to clear.

- Don't eat right before going to bed. Your body needs to digest the food, which interferes with sleep (and my mom says it gives you nightmares).

- Make time to actually watch the end of the sunset and keep the lights dim before bedtime. This initiates melatonin production and makes you sleepy.

- Cut out the evening caffeine. It's a stimulant that messes up your sleep cycles and causes your nervous system to be in an excited state.

- Don't keep a TV in the bedroom, watch TV, or look at a computer screen at least an hour before bedtime. The light stimulates an awakened state.

- Regulate your circadian rhythm by going to bed at the same time each night. Make a nightly habit of relaxing, reading, and praying to prepare your body for sleep.

- Keep naps to the suggested 15- to 30-minute length. Longer than this can interfere with your body's ability to fall and stay asleep.

HOW MUCH SLEEP DO WE NEED?

We all know that we need sleep, but how much do we really need? Of course, it depends on the age of the person. The number of hours of sleep to be fully recharged can also depend on the person's activity level and health level. All of us need more when we're sick or fatigued. Here's a table showing recommended amounts based on several major sleep organizations.

Sleep Table

Stage	Age	Minimum (in hours)	Normal Amt. (in hours)	Maximum (in hours)
Elderly	≥65 years	5	7-8	9
Adult	26-64 years	6	7-9	10
Young Adult	18-25 years	6	7-9	11
Teenager	13-17 years	7	8-10	11
Child	6-12 years	8	9-11	12
Preschooler	3-5 years	9	10-13	14
Toddler	1-2 years	10	11-14	16
Infant	4-11 mos.	11	12-15	18
Newborn	0-3 mos.	12	14-17	19

I'm always surprised by patients who seem to be confused by the fact that they're feeling the need to have *more* sleep than usual when they're experiencing pain in their bodies or when they're sick. Having grown up in a health-centered family, it was obvious to me that when I was injured or fighting an illness, my body was going to require more rest to repair itself or fight infection. I assumed everyone knew this, but apparently not. So, let me make it clear. If you're tired and feeling sleepy…go to bed. Your body is trying to tell you something and your health depends on it!

Another area concerning the quantity of sleep that's often overlooked involves the effect of emotional health on the amount of sleep that you need. Emotional stress takes a tremendous toll on the amount of energy and resources that the body uses to maintain balance. Anyone who's been extremely stressed out (which is all of us at times), can tell you that they can become exhausted in a short period of time. Research tells us that when people are made to perform more complicated or difficult mental tasks, they burn more energy by increased cellular function throughout the body, but especially in the brain.

The challenge with emotional strain, or what most of us simply call stress, is that it can affect us all day long, even if we're not consciously thinking about something. This causes us to become tired throughout the day and have little reserves to be able to handle whatever comes next.

The bottom line with how much sleep you need is that, in most cases, your body will tell you when you've had enough sleep. If you've had several relaxing days on vacation and you begin waking up feeling refreshed after only seven hours of sleep, then that's probably all you need. On the other hand, if after eight hours of sleep your alarm clock, or a marching band for that matter, can't wake you up, then I'm gonna go out on a limb here and say that you might need just a little bit more sleep. Ya think?

HOW TO GET MORE SLEEP

So, how *do* we actually get more sleep? I know this sounds obvious and simplistic, but one key is to simply set a time to go to bed and actually stop what you're doing in time to get ready and be in bed by your set time.

The truth is we can't get around the fact that we all have 24 hours in a day. You've got to draw a **hard line** and define the time that you will absolutely stop everything and get ready for bed. Take one night and time yourself when you're getting ready for bed. Start timing from the moment you turn off the TV, or the computer, or whatever you're doing, and stop timing when you've actually set your alarm clock, turned out the lights, and closed your eyes. Remember that this time of "getting ready for bed" includes feeding the dog, getting clothes or food ready for the next day, finishing the last few dishes in the sink, washing your face, brushing your teeth, end-of-the-day stretches, saying your prayers, or anything else you do every night before you go to bed.

Now that you have that time estimated, count backward from the time you want to go to bed, and that's when you start getting ready. For example, if you determine that it takes you 30 minutes to get ready for bed, and that you want to go to bed at 10 o'clock, then you need to start getting ready at 9:30. It's actually pretty simple. We can choose to go to bed on time or stay up later than we intended.

Either way we slice it, we'll pay the piper. If we stay up late, we'll be tired and cranky, weaken our immune system, diminish our reserves, and possibly even get sick. If we go to bed on time and choose not to watch one more important episode of *Redneck Truckers in Alaska*, the consequence is that we won't get to discuss it at the water cooler tomorrow. Hmm, you decide which consequence is worse.

Have you ever heard that if you miss some sleep, you can't make it up? That's just flat-out not true. You *have* to make it up. By not getting enough sleep, you now have a deficit that will be made up by your body in one way or another. You'll be tired and drag for several days or weeks until you nap and sleep enough to get back to normal. Your body can't be fooled, and you can't make up sleep while functioning at normal capacity. As you're reading this, you may be functioning at a substandard level because you have a cumulative deficit of sleep that's been building for several weeks, months, or even years.

There's all kinds of research that shows how poorly athletes, students, employees, truck drivers, and pretty much anyone who doesn't get enough sleep, performs the activities set before them. Mistakes can be extremely costly, depending on what activity you're doing. Would you like a neurosurgeon, who is short on sleep, to cut you open and perform brain surgery? Me neither. How about airline pilots, dentists, or even the guy at the crosswalk at your kid's school? We're all designed to be rested, sharp, thinking clearly, and ready to tackle anything that life brings our way.

NAPPING

This is one often overlooked part of rest that's important to discuss. Many people even joke about how they wish they could take a nap but never consider it seriously. If Thomas Edison and Albert Einstein thought it was a good idea to do regularly, then that's good enough for me.[5]

When you're a kid, you're forced to nap and you fight it kicking and screaming. When you grow up, however, you really want to take one, but the boss won't let you—so not fair! What's really funny is that numerous studies show how much increased efficiency and focus you have when refreshed from a midday nap…you'd actually be more productive. The body is already naturally experiencing "post-prandial stupor" (doctor talk for being sleepy after eating), so it's the obvious time to take a little snooze.

Harvard reported that taking a short afternoon nap can improve learning, memory, and creative thinking without interfering with your nighttime sleep schedule or pattern.[6] I also recently read several reports from Japan that explained how many companies had their employees take a "power" nap of 20–30 minutes after eating lunch. Some made it mandatory, turned off the phones, computers, machinery and lights, and even provided mats for the workers to lie down on and rest. The research found a significant decrease in mistakes after the power nap in only a few short weeks of instituting the new rule. They actually worked less total time in the week, but performance increased during those hours.[7]

Maybe more employers should require a nap instead of punishing people for taking one. Studies have also found that employees who nap were happier with their jobs and had fewer missed work days due to illnesses. I personally recommend that my staff members nap each day at lunchtime. Aren't they lucky? What I recommend then, if you're at work, is to find a quiet, comfortable spot, possibly in your car, and get a 15–30 minute nap each day. The flatter you can lie, the better.

When I lived over an hour away from work, I would drive to a local park just around the corner from my office and park under a shade tree after lunch. I'd put the seat all the way back and crack the windows and "saw some logs." On cold days, I'd park in the sun. It's amazing how the sun can heat you up, even on a cold day.

To get a "power nap" you have to get serious and turn off your phone and all other distractions that could wake you.

If you're at home, then obviously your bed is the ideal place to lie horizontally and stretch out. Try resting on your back, on a neck roll or a curved pillow so that you support the normal "rainbow curve" in your neck. Even if you don't normally sleep in this position, it's great for your body and many people can do it quite well for short periods of time. This will help stretch out the neck and upper back that has likely been slouching all day while at your work station.

Some people can nap sitting in a chair, but this is *not* recommended. When you sleep in a chair, you tend to slouch, stressing the low back. The head also hangs forward, which puts stress on the neck and upper back. This contributes to forward head posture, a "Dowagers hump," and all kinds of degeneration, pain, bone spurs, and even compression fractures in the spine.

To get a "power nap" you have to get serious and turn off your phone and all other distractions that could wake you. Try turning on some "white noise" to block out the other sounds around you. If you need to, set an alarm to wake you at an appropriate time. In the end, napping will absolutely increase your level of health. I'm positive that it's part of the Original Design for health.

SLEEP AIDS

If you're having trouble sleeping, then ask your doctor or nutritionist about taking natural or herbal sleep aids. There are many different natural remedies that can be and have been used in traditional cultures for thousands of years. Please try these before using addictive drugs.

One simple place to start is with minerals. Minerals have a tranquilizing effect on most people and can calm you down significantly while supplying nutrients that your body may be in need of anyway. Always try to go with an organic, food-sourced mineral supplement instead of hard-to-absorb "rock dust" that comes from a nonorganic chemical source. Some naturally mineral-rich foods are algae, sea kelp, and many green leafy vegetables. The old wife's tale of warm milk to help you sleep may be due to the minerals in the milk, including calcium, but it also may be due to the good fats.

Melatonin is a hormone that's produced by the pineal gland in the brain and is your body's natural form of "sleepy juice." Many companies re-create this substance synthetically in the lab or from "natural plant and/or animal sources," and sell it as a sleep aid in an oral spray (quickly absorbed) or pill form. From a strictly herbal standpoint, there are many substances that can be useful in inducing drowsiness. A short list includes valerian, chamomile, passion flower, kava kava, and California poppy. Some preparations will include several of them mixed together to create a supertonic of synergistic compounds.

Liquid herbal extracts, capsules or dry tablet forms are the typical way that these substances are found commercially. Research the brand or company that you purchase from first, as potency and compound bioactivity vary widely from seller to seller. (There's more on this in the supplement chapter.)

From there, we get into drugs or medicine. Over-the-counter sleep-aids or painkiller PM pills and liquids usually have Diphenhydramine HCL as the active ingredient used to create drowsiness. Just so you know, in case you have any sensitivity, that drug is also known as Benadryl, which has an antihistamine effect too. Always check with your doctor to choose wisely and to make sure there are no contraindications to taking over-the-counter medications along with your prescriptions.

You can also ask your doctor about prescription medications to help you sleep, but in my opinion they should be a last resort. Many of them can be extremely addictive and have a whole host of unpleasant side effects associated with them. Additionally, they cover up symptoms that may be stemming from a much deeper psychological or health condition. It's always a better idea to try and determine what your problem is before you start taking a medication that will only mask a symptom and not get to the heart of the issue. There are certain genetic conditions or periods of time in life that, for a short while, may require medication.

This is where the benefits of medication are extremely apparent, and we should be thankful that we have the medical profession to help us at these times. However, the vast majority of the time, with stress reduction, exercise, good spinal alignment, prayer, diet modification, natural supplements, and the other tips in the list above, you can regain the restful sleep you were originally designed to have without dangerous medications.

It's part of the Original Design for our bodies and minds to have plentiful rest. I'd encourage you to begin to get the sleep you need and allow your body to restore itself through much-needed and highly beneficial rest.

PILLAR III

CHEMICAL

CHAPTER 11

DIET

This is the longest chapter of the book for one simple reason: There's so much confusion and difference of opinion about diet. Innumerable volumes of books have been written on the subject that will tell you exactly what you should eat. Who are you supposed to believe? It's overwhelming! Aren't you glad I'm here to make it easy? ☺

I saw a PBS special several years ago called *Diet Wars* that was a debate between some of the most influential nutrition experts in the US. It was sponsored by the USDA. Dr. Atkins was proposing a high-protein and high-fat diet, Dr. Ornish was proposing a high-carbohydrate and low-fat diet, and Dr. Sears, who published the *Zone Diet*, was proposing a balance of fat, protein, and carbs equally, and several other doctors, all with differing opinions. They started off politely but then began to raise their voices toward the other panelists, even going so far as to stand up and point fingers while yelling at each other! Needless to say, it got just a tad bit heated. They all felt very strongly about their stance on nutrition and none of them were willing to back down one inch.

While I was watching, a lightbulb went off in my mind, and I had one of those "duh" moments. What hit me was that all of these doctors had documented results of helping patients, and yet they all achieved it differently. While none of them could agree on carbs, fats, and proteins, they all recommended cutting out processed junk foods and adding significantly more fresh fruits and vegetables. It kinda makes you wonder if those just might be the two *most* important things after all. Now that's "food for thought." (Pun intended.)

We were designed to eat and thrive on the foods that God designed, put on the earth, and made readily available.

Here's the deal: I'm pretty sure I've never heard two doctors, nutritionists, dieticians, or health experts of any kind agree on diet. I'm sure I'll hear plenty of negative remarks about *my* ideas too. People love to tell you what they think...especially with social media these days. That's okay, because we're all entitled to our opinions. The funny thing is, based on research, many opinions can and will change. The scientific community is constantly learning and reevaluating what they believe.

That being said, the solid foundational principles of the Original Design Diet will *never* change. These principles are based on God's design, the history of the human race, science, and common sense and will help you easily navigate through the world of diet and nutrition.

My core belief about what we eat and the main guiding principle to understanding an ideal diet is simple and it's wrapped up in the basic idea of the Original Design. We were designed to eat and thrive on the foods that God designed, put on the earth, and made readily available. Each of the foods that we were given have value and play their own unique role in creating a healthy body. That hasn't changed, and it never will. The design remains the same to this day and forevermore.

In fact, research suggests that, overall, our basic DNA is practically unchanged since the beginning of mankind. This means that our dietary needs are practically unchanged as well. From the beginning, we humans regularly drank good amounts of clean water to quench our thirst. We've always consumed proteins and nearly equal amounts of omega-6 and omega-3 fats[1] in the form of fish and other seafood, animals and their dairy products, and birds and their eggs, which also contain saturated and monounsaturated fats.

In addition, we've consistently eaten nutrient-dense and antioxidant-rich foods from plants like nuts, seeds, properly prepared grains, beans, vegetables, and fruits that provide healthy and valuable carbohydrates and fiber. Along with those naturally occurring foods are countless micronutrients like enzymes, coenzymes, probiotics, phytonutrients, and other cofactors, some of which are yet to be discovered, but we need them all and they've *always existed* in those foods according to the Original Design.

Random side note: An animal out in nature, eating what it was designed to eat and living as it was designed to live, doesn't need to see a veterinarian. Once you take it outside out of its natural habitat and feed it engineered food, it often gets sick, gains too much weight and becomes diseased. Sound familiar?

Anyway, as time has gone on, we've created more industrialized societies and we've begun to damage our food supply. Through industrial processing, heavy chemical usage, and genetic engineering, we've created foods that aren't only deficient in these valuable nutrients, but they can cause major issues for normal digestion, allergies, severe fatigue, and diseases, like autoimmune problems, cardiovascular disease, and even cancer.

NICK'S STORY

I'm reminded of one of my patients who overheard me counseling another patient one day about her child's diet and its connection to allergies and digestive issues. She asked me a few questions and the very the next week we began to work with her son who was having awful problems. Here's her son's story in her words:

Nicholas is my third son. My first two sons were healthy, happy babies. Nicholas was happy until about four months of age. At that time, he started to be very fussy and cried most of the time when he was awake. He had eczema all over his body and even prominently on his face.

He was often very congested and wheezy. The doctor diagnosed him with asthma and suggested steroid-based breathing treatments multiple times a day. We were opposed to steroids for a baby so we looked for alternatives. We tried to see allergists but they would *not* see him because his skin was scaly and broken out—they wouldn't be able to test him.

We took him to specialists and months went by. We did breathing treatments when he was particularly bad. No one had answers. By 14 months of age, he'd had a series of lung infections including RSV and was still crying for hours, day after day. We were desperate to know what was wrong with our baby. He looked sickly all of the time with dark circles under his swollen eyes and blotchy, red, dry skin. He didn't smile, had a chronically runny nose, bags under his eyes, a rattling chest cough, he cried constantly and barely played with his brothers.

One day I went to see Dr. Mark for my appointment and Nicholas was with me. He suggested that Nicholas might be suffering from food allergies and that we consider altering his diet to consist of only organic fruits, vegetables, and organic meats. I was skeptical but willing to try anything. We altered his diet *that* day.

Three days later I picked him up from his home day care and for the first time I could remember, Nicholas smiled…and I cried. His skin was clear, his tummy was no longer hard and distended, and he was happy! Within seven days, all the symptoms, including the cough, were gone! More than half of his life had been spent being miserable.

After that, Nicholas became a happy baby and has grown into a happy, healthy young boy! He has gluten intolerance and we discovered that the baby puffs (along with tons of other foods) that I was feeding him starting at three months contained wheat and gluten, which his body can't process. He was cramping and in pain all the time, and that resulted in the constant crying. Thank you, Dr. Mark—you're still our hero!

I love that story and it proves an important point: We've strayed way too far from the Original Design for the diet that our bodies are designed to thrive on and it's had devastating consequences. It's time for us to refocus on what we're eating and drinking and get back on the original path.

It can't be rocket science to figure out what to eat, or humans would've starved to death thousands of years ago and we wouldn't even be here today.

IT WAS DESIGNED TO BE EASY

Another guiding principle about diet that's important to understand has to do with determining *what* our diet should be. It can't be rocket science to figure out what to eat, or humans would've starved to death thousands of years ago and we wouldn't even be here today. The problem is that we've way overcomplicated things. Think about it. If finding and preparing nutritious food that was designed to nourish our bodies was extremely difficult, then considering our propensity for laziness, we'd all be "toast." Instead, people have *thrived*, and in widely varying environments too.

These originally designed foods were also meant to be in great abundance worldwide. While the foods may have varied, they were available on all of the continents and islands that people have traditionally lived. No matter where humans lived, there were nearly always readily available and healthy sources of water, good fats, proteins, carbohydrates, and all the other micronutrients, some that may yet be discovered.

We'll get into greater detail as we go along, but let me state it simply with a purposefully and ridiculously long run-on sentence: Do you really think it's a coincidence that an animal, like a cow, which has hundreds of pounds of nourishing fats and proteins and vitamins and minerals and enzymes and cofactors in its meat and dairy products, and whose meat tastes and smells so amazingly good when cooked over a fire, moves incredibly slow and isn't real bright or capable of avoiding being easily captured and used as a plentiful source of healthy food (and other raw materials)? Nope. God designed it to be easy.

This reminds me of hiding Easter eggs for my kids when they were just two or three years old. I'd put their eggs out in the open where they were easy to find. I'm their father and I love them—I didn't make the eggs ridiculously hard to find. What kind of father would do that? We only did that for their teenage cousins! ☺

We could also liken this to the convenience and nourishment available to babies from their mother's milk. God intended nutrition to be simple, obvious, and enjoyable. Babies don't have to look very far for the most nutritious and delicious meal that their bodies were designed to thrive on. Mommy is holding them closely, and lunch is right there. The baby doesn't have to research, read a book, attend a seminar, or do anything complicated—it's *designed* to be easy. Follow me?

Imagine that you're walking through the forest and you see a small red thing growing on a plant that catches your eye in the distance on the forest floor. You notice that it's beautiful to the eye, and so you walk over to it, pick it, and find that it's amazingly fragrant to the nose. When you taste it, you realize it's sweet, juicy, and full of unbelievable flavor. Isn't it obvious that there's a design or purpose in that? Of course there is! Recognizing it as food is part of our Original Design. In fact, not only is it delicious but it's also incredibly good for you. It's designed to be full of a wide array of crucial nutrients that your body needs to function normally and healthily.

The problem comes in, of course, when we begin to alter the foods that were originally designed for us to eat, and chemically process and alter or "engineer" them. They become "food-like substances" that may *taste* okay initially, but in fact they're unhealthy for our bodies. They're deceptive counterfeits of the real thing. In Texas, this is what we call "no bueno."

By the way, isn't that really similar to how counterfeit ways to live that *seem* right in the beginning, in actuality, lead to problems that alter our lives from the Original Design and rob us of health in the end? Like how staying out late, partying, getting drunk, and getting very little sleep seems like a great idea at first, (when you're in college) but then not so much in the morning?

GOOD MOTIVES GONE WRONG

Before we go any further, let's agree on something: The bottom line of all industry is what? Every time I ask this question when I'm speaking at a conference, the entire audience says the exact same word—so say it with me: The bottom line of all industry is...*money*. We all know that money drives all industry because of the simple fact that, in our society, we have to have it to survive, so let's keep that in mind.

What I don't want to do is confuse you about my opinion of the *motives* of the people who work for large corporations in the food industry. The majority of people working in the food industry are normal, goodhearted people who are simply trying to make a living to provide for their families.

Take, for instance, the first inventors of food additives and preservatives. As populations grew, especially in cities where there were dense populations of people in a small area, the problem of food spoilage became quite prevalent. Since people had limited access to fresh foods in these cities, they relied on grocers to ship it to them from the farmers in the country. This presented a challenge for the industry to come up with a way to keep food on the shelves longer without going bad.

In my opinion, they honestly began to experiment with techniques and substances that would meet this need. As they did so, and the technology increased, more and more chemicals became available. Little did they know that the road they were going down was going to be a disaster for the health of all humanity. We now have the results of that, which is a packaged, engineered food supply that's focused more on its ability to have a long shelf life, look good, taste good, and have maximum profit for companies, than anything having to do with improving or maintaining our health.

What we all know is that when we sacrifice quality for price, we're often not happy with what we get, especially in the long term. Again, I don't believe that these engineers intended to malnourish our population and create cancer-causing "fake foods" that would cause the demise of the human race. However, we're unfortunately well on our way in that direction.

International research points to chemical exposure in various forms as being one of the greatest causes of degenerative conditions, including cardiovascular disease, diabetes, obesity, and cancer, as well as even things like infertility and mental issues. There are, of course, other factors that contribute to these health disasters, but there is good reason to believe that chemicals, industrial processing, and genetic engineering are major factors. Okay, now on to what we *should* put in our bodies.

WATER

Before we get into food, we need to discuss the single most critical factor and common denominator of the diets, nutrition, and health of every culture throughout the world: H2O. Every group of humans throughout history, from small nomadic tribes to massive civilizations, have made finding a clean, steady source of water their number-one priority. As an amateur archaeologist, I've studied early cultures of humans around the globe, and it quickly becomes clear that they all settled near a stream, river, lake, or spring where clean water could be easily and regularly secured.

Water is critical to human survival. Roughly 70% of our bodies are made of water. We can only live for three to five days without it, whereas we can live three to five weeks without food. Water is necessary for the normal functioning of every cell in your body.

The challenge in our modern world is that most people don't drink enough water. I've had countless patients whose health improved dramatically when they simply began to drink more water on a regular basis. That's simple medicine. One doctor I heard of won't even begin to treat a patient until he or she is getting adequate water intake. This is because he found that a large percentage of people's health issues "magically" disappear when they get enough water in their system. Imagine that!

There's no mystery as to why water tastes so good when you're thirsty. We were originally designed to *need* water and to yearn to drink it. It wasn't until cultures were more advanced that they regularly drank other beverages for their daily water requirement.

I remember one patient in particular who came in for nutritional counseling. I asked him, "How much water have you had to drink today?" He said, "Well, I had two cups of coffee this morning, part of a can of diet cola at lunch, a small energy drink on the way here, and...uh...I think that's it." It was five o'clock! Immediately, I knew where to start with him. We can't get by on that little liquid! When we don't get enough water, we begin to have common symptoms like "thirst, dry mouth, dry skin, dry nose which can lead to nosebleeds, fatigue, nausea, headaches, dizziness, rapid heart rate, loss of appetite, weakness, dark yellow urine and infrequent urination,"[2] to name a few.

My dad always says that his drill sergeant in the military used to say, "If you're not peeing clear, you're not drinking enough!" Hydration is adequate when you're urinating every two to four hours that you're awake, or six to eight times per day, eliminating one to two quarts of water daily,[3] and the color is clear to light yellow.

A good rule of thumb for how much water to drink is half your body weight in ounces. So if you weigh 170 pounds, then you should drink about 85 ounces of water, or 2.5 liters, which is five standard 16.9 ounce bottles. We've got to stay hydrated!

The next question is always, what kind of water should I drink? There's a ton of debate on this subject, and I'll simply say that getting water as close to its Original Design, like from a spring, is ideal. Researchers disagree and cases can be made for alkaline mineral water, rainwater, reverse osmosis, filtered, and glacial melt-off, etc. I'd personally be most concerned with avoiding plastic contaminants like PVCs and phthalates, pathogenic bacteria, parasites, and chemicals like fluoride and chlorine. Do your own personal research, but don't get too worried about it. Stress can ruin your health faster than a little dirt in your water.

A good rule of thumb for how much water to drink is half your body weight in ounces.

I LOVE TO EAT

Let's move on to diet. This is certainly one of my favorite subjects because I love to eat. I think I probably got this from my mother, who also loves to eat and enjoys flavors of all kinds. My mom is an amazing cook and was the one who gave me basic kitchen smarts; she taught me how to make nearly every bit of food that I can make. She also gave me the love for preparing, sharing, and eating food as well.

I did happen to watch a few cooking shows along the way too (back when I actually did have some spare time and only four channels of TV). I watched chefs like the Ragin' Cajun, Justin Wilson, the French gourmand, Jacques Pepin, and later on, the BAM! master, Emeril Lagasse. It was Mom, though, who first taught me that things always taste better when they're homemade and when the ingredients are fresh. Growing up, it was fun to use ingredients like herbs and vegetables from our garden. In fact, I don't ever remember a time when my mom made spaghetti sauce by dumping a prepared jar of some factory-made glop into the skillet. She always started with fresh ingredients and made it, and all of her sauces and dishes, from scratch.

Subsequently, I knew the difference between the flavor of real mashed potatoes and powdered, the difference between fresh and canned vegetables, and the difference between real and fake ingredients. I think the only time I ever ate a frozen "TV dinner" was in college when I was swamped with studying. Seriously, it was straight-up nasty. I figured I was making the sacrifice with food to get the grade I was shooting for. I was wrong.

I didn't do that again, and I continued to cook my own meals. It tasted better and was healthier for me—I knew it because of how I had been raised. As you might imagine, word spread that I was whippin' up some good ole home cookin', and it wasn't surprising to have an apartment full of friends on any given night. Moochers.

Back to growing up, even though we loved mom's fresh-baked bread, it was a rarity and so bread carbs typically were kept to a minimum. Dessert, however, was always a constant. She baked pies, cakes, cookies, lemon squares, and brownies. My mom contributed her sweet-tooth gene to my DNA, I'm afraid. The key was that it was homemade with natural ingredients, and that we only had a *small* serving.

PORTION CONTROL AND LOSING WEIGHT

Mom taught us that you could please your mouth, nose, and tummy with a variety of ever-changing flavors, but you didn't have to gorge yourself to feel good and enjoy what you were eating. In fact, it was stuffing yourself that actually diminished your overall culinary experience, usually created stomach pain, and caused you to gain weight.

I clearly remember going to Thanksgiving with my extended family of usually 75 folks or so when I was a kid, and having a dessert plate that was as big as my entrée plate. This idea might sound a little gluttonous, but we only did it a few times a year and I rarely ate it all. I believe it's actually a key to happy, healthy eating habits.

My mom taught me that you could cut pieces of pie or cookies in half or quarters to sample all the tastes that my talented Polish family members had spent so much time making from scratch in their own kitchens. Make your taste buds sing with variety and flavors, just don't drown them or stuff yourself. This started in the entrée side of the meal, in that we had several different veggies and a salad, so we had to eat smaller helpings of things to get them all in. We were expected to eat what we took, so Mom taught us to start out small and get more if we were still hungry.

Notice that she taught us only to get more *if* we were still hungry. One of the main challenges with obesity and diet in America is quantity. It's fairly simple: If you weigh too much, you're eating more than your body can use. People are totally unaware of how few calories it actually takes to thrive, not just survive. When I discuss with patients the quantity of food or the total number of calories to eat every day, many of them seem surprised at how little I'm suggesting they eat. We've been programmed incorrectly by our society. People *think* they need more food than they actually do. Like my mom taught me, our girls know to stop when their tummy tells them to.

Now before y'all start shooting at me, I realize, of course, that there are differences in genetics and that it's harder for some people to lose or gain weight. I have close friends in both of those categories, so I completely understand. Either way, it just takes time.

There was a patient of mine who started eating right, exercising, and getting adjusted. We really worked hard to work through some challenges and get her on a good path. She came in one day after about three weeks after sticking closely to her plan, and she said, "I'm so disappointed…I've only lost three pounds!" I reminded her that there were 52 weeks in a year and that if she kept up this simple plan, she'd lose 52 pounds in one year. A year and a half later, she'd lost about 65 pounds, had little to no pain, and hadn't felt that good since she was a kid!

Of course, exercise increases your metabolism too. However, the principle still holds true that how much and what you eat has a great deal to do with determining your weight, but more importantly, your level of health. Diet always comes down to these two issues: quantity and quality.

Quantity is easy to understand. To put it plainly, when you see pictures of the horrible conditions in the concentration camps of Nazi Germany, you realize that everyone was starving and unbelievably thin, to the point of ribs and pelvic bones showing. These people barely had enough food to stay alive. In fact, tragically, many died because they didn't have enough food. On the extreme other end of the spectrum, you'll see TV shows about people with eating disorders who weigh over 500 pounds. Clearly, they are eating way more than their bodies can ever use, and so the excess calories are stored as fat.

The obvious conclusion is that there's a happy medium for each of us individually for the total amount of calories that we need to thrive on, so that we're not starving *or* morbidly obese. It takes some experimentation to figure out, but you'll find that you'll do just fine on half a sandwich or one enchilada instead of two. It all depends on your body type, age, sex, genetics, and activity level. You're unique and what's healthy for you won't necessarily be healthy for someone else, nor will you "look" like others. There's an Original Design that is specific to you.

We need to renew our minds to what "healthy" looks like. When you see a fitness magazine cover, you're not necessarily seeing ideal health; rather, you're seeing someone who has focused only on eliminating body fat but may have done so in an unhealthy way. Many times those pictures are taken after days of starvation and severe water restrictions. That's not realistic.

Quality of our diet is a little more complex. But keeping in mind what I said above, I believe that what we eat was designed to be fairly easy to figure out. Overall, we need to eat foods that are as close to their Original Design as possible. In the end, if we eat the whole, organic, unprocessed foods that God designed for us to eat, then we'll get the health we were designed to have. When we eat engineered, chemical-laden junk foods, we become unhealthy, which was not the Original Design.

"GRABBING A BITE"

How we eat is also something to consider. When we eat meals at the table, as we always did growing up, with the whole family, we take a little more time to eat. There was a relaxed atmosphere, laughter, and conversation, which is conducive to eating a little more slowly and therefore promoting good digestion.

When you eat slower, your body has a chance to send the "stop eating, silly, you're full!" messages to your brain, and you end up eating less. Stuffing food in the "pie hole" is not good. When we're rushed or stressed out while eating, we stimulate the "fight or flight" part of our autonomic nervous system known as the sympathetic nervous system. This system gets us ready for "strenuous muscle actions," and it also has the temporary side effect of slowing down or even shutting off our digestive systems.

Is it any wonder that we have the digestive problems we do in this country when so many Americans are eating on the go, in a hurry, in their cars, at fast-food restaurants, or quickly before the next event in their busy day? Often, people eat while arguing with a family member or watching a violent or adrenaline-pumping TV show. Patients frequently tell me they need to get something to eat really quickly and say things like, "I'm just going to *grab* a bite on the way to the...."

How about we turn off the overload to our sympathetic nervous system and sit down with relaxing music or even this crazy thing called silence while we enjoy a meal with our family? Who knows, we might actually talk to each other. We might just see some significant improvement in our personal peace, digestive health, family unity, and happiness. Sound good? It does to me too.

YOU ARE WHAT YOU EAT...*AND* WHAT IT ATE

I was watching an episode of *The Cat in the Hat* on PBS with my kids one morning before I began to write. They were talking about flamingos and how their babies are white, but as they begin to grow, they turn pink. They went on to say that the pink color is from the algae that they eat. That's not *exactly* correct. They skipped a step or two. The pink color actually comes from astaxanthin, which is a carotenoid that has a pink color to it. It's much like another carotenoid, beta-carotene, which gives carrots their orange color.

Astaxanthin in particular is created by sunlight exposure to certain types of algae in the ocean. Little crustaceans like brine shrimp, which are called zooplankton, then eat the algae, thereby depositing the astaxanthin in their bodies and shells. After flamingos eat these little critters, the pink color is deposited in *their* feathers and skin. Needless to say, they didn't explain all of that on the cartoon, but I had to tell my kids. Sorry—it's the science geek in me. I have to admit, I'm not quite sure that our three-year-old got all of what I said.

The point is that understanding the food chain is crucial. It's incredibly important to know what the diet was of the bird, fish, or animal that you're eating. This is absolutely critical for our health. Take a look at the chart below to get an idea of what I mean.

The Original Design Food Chain

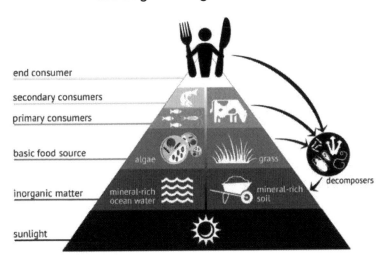

Let's take salmon, for example. Wild baby salmon eat algae and plankton, and as they get older they eat shrimp, krill, and small fish that eat plankton too. This nutrient-dense and astaxanthin-rich diet gives their flesh or "meat" the pink color. Their meat has roughly 60% more omega-3 fat, 15% more protein and 27% less total fat than farm-raised salmon.[4]

Sadly, farm-raised salmon don't get these naturally nutrient-dense foods. They're fed a man-made feed pellet that can come from GMO soy and GMO corn meal, as well as by-products of other industries and chemical residues that were *never* designed to be food for them. Therefore, synthetic astaxanthin (which is not approved for human consumption) has to be added to the feed to give salmon the pink color that people expect.[5] What? That's crazy! I've actually seen "color added" on a salmon label in the fish department of a grocery store. Lawsuits have even been filed against grocery chains that failed to label these fish as having chemicals added.[6]

The obvious problem is that when you eat the salmon that is given fake "foods" that they weren't designed to eat, then you're eating a food that *you* weren't designed to eat. Their diet was deficient and chemical tainted and now...so is yours!

There's an incredibly important and foundational truth here: It's not just about what you eat but how and where what you eat was raised and what it ate before getting to your dinner plate. This is critical to the concept of the Original Design Diet.

The poor treatment, diet, and living conditions of stock animals like cattle, confinement factory-raised chicken, and farm-raised fish has been a popular cause recently. Proper conditions aren't just an added bonus for the mental and physical health of the animal, bird, or fish, but it's critical for your health as well.

For instance, let's look at eggs. It's not enough for me to just make a vague statement and say that eggs are good for you. The kind of eggs makes a huge difference. We used to be told that eggs were good for us. Anyone remember "♫The incredible, edible egg!♫" commercials? Then "they" decided that eggs weren't good for us—all that cholesterol (not true, by the way!). Then they said that you could eat egg whites for the protein, but to throw away the yolks because they would "clog your arteries." How ridiculous is that? (Wait till you read the section on cholesterol in my next book—your body actually needs it!)

One study "examined the relation between egg consumption and incidence of CHD (coronary heart disease) and stroke in a cohort of 80,082 women 34 through 59 years of age…and found no evidence of an…association between egg consumption and risk of CHD." In fact, their research showed a slight *decrease* in risk when they ate five to six eggs per week.[7]

Pasture-raised eggs come from chickens that live out in nature, in the fresh air and sunshine, and eat bugs, worms, grass, seeds, nuts, and plants… what they were *designed* to eat. These birds will create eggs that are valuable, dense sources of nutrients that we need, like protein, good cholesterol, omega-3 fats, vitamins A and E, beta-carotene, and choline to just name a few. When consumed during pregnancy, choline, which is found in the yoke, has even been shown to reduce neural tube defects in babies.[8] This type of eggs is extremely healthy for your body. It might be the perfect food.

Conventional (cheap) eggs come from chickens that are confined in a warehouse, standing shoulder to shoulder with thousands of other chickens, and will not produce the healthy eggs that you and your loved ones need and deserve. The living conditions of these birds are atrocious. They're often made to stand "knee-deep" in their own urine and feces, without access to sunlight, grass, or fresh air...ever. Many have painful skin conditions, respiratory problems, pulmonary congestion, swelling, hemorrhaging, and blindness from the ammonia gases coming off of their waste. They're frequently diseased or even die before harvesting.[9]

They're fed a diet of man-made pellets of processed GMO soy, GMO cottonseed, GMO canola, feather meal, and various other industries' waste products and contain chemical residues, like antibiotics and even Prozac.[10] 70% of these chickens have arsenic added to their feed as it's thought to help with disease and give the meat a nice pink color.[11] This is unbelievable and not even remotely close to the Original Design.

Let's look at the differences in the wording on egg cartons, how they're raised and how that affects the nutrition of the eggs. Here are the main types you'll find in the grocery store:

- Pasture-raised: Original Design eggs (see above).

- Conventional: raised in a barn (see above).

- Omega-3: still conventional but given omega-3 "enriched" feed.

- Cage-free: still conventional and while not in cages, they're still in big barns.

- Free-range: still conventional, but with a small access door to a little dirt patch.

- Organic: still conventional, not given hormones or antibiotics, fed an organic pellet, but *not* pastured.

Here are some potential nutrient differences:

Nutrients per 100 g. of egg	Vitamin A (IU)	Vitamin E (mg)	Vitamin D[12] (IU)	Beta-carotene (mcg)	Omega-3 (g)
Conventional[13]	487	.97	35	10	.22
Pasture-raised[14]	1013	4.02	210	100	.74

The pasture-raised eggs have roughly two times the vitamin A, four times the vitamin E, six times the vitamin D, ten times the beta-carotene, and three and a half times the omega-3s! Still worried about cost? I think they're *worth* a little more than the conventional eggs, don't you? The taste is even better too. They're what eggs were designed to be like before the chickens' diets and lifestyles were so drastically changed from the Original Design. Am I getting through yet?

While we can't control the quality of foods when we eat out, we must ensure that all the foods that we buy for home preparation are as close to their Original Design as possible. When animals, fish, or birds are raised the way they were designed to live, it ensures that they and their products are full of the nutrients that we were designed to thrive on. Furthermore, they also won't be genetically modified or contain hormones, antibiotics, pesticides, herbicides, fungicides, or other chemicals that can harm you and your family.

This also applies to what you buy in the produce section. The soil that fruits and veggies are grown in determines what's inside of them. Nutrient-depleted soils yield fruits and vegetables with depleted nutrients like vitamins and minerals. Therefore, you don't get the nutrients you need from produce grown in those soils that could leave you susceptible to various deficiencies and illnesses. This is why buying or growing organic produce is so important. Our very health is dependent on the rules of the Original Design being applied to all aspects of food, whether it's an animal or a plant.

ORGANIC

A study came out recently that was supposed to have once and for all debunked the myth that organic produce is of greater value than conventional or nonorganic produce. I spent hours over the following weeks with patients who brought it up, trying to explain why that "study" was completely ridiculous.

Where do I start? Okay, first off, let's go back to a guiding principle of this book: The further we get away from what God designed, the bigger our problems get. The Original Design for any food is the ideal for our bodies. Keeping that in mind, the term *organic*, by law, means that it's not genetically modified, synthetic pesticide and herbicide-free, nonirradiated, hormone and antibiotic-free. That sounds like the Original Design to me. At least it's closer than conventional produce.

There are many studies showing a reduction of chemicals in the human bloodstream when eating organic, but one in particular sticks out. Funded by the EPA, this recent study, which was performed by researchers from Emory University, the University of Washington, and the CDC, had startling results. They tested the blood of children who ate conventional foods and found the presence of multiple chemicals. In comparison, blood samples from the same children after they had switched to eating all organic versions of the same foods showed that the levels dropped to near nondetectable levels.[15]

We need to be conscious of the foods that we eat and the products that we use in order to avoid chemicals that are potentially dangerous to our health. These chemicals are not part of the Original Design and routinely are found to cause everything from common illnesses to cancer. More issues are being found daily. Organic is the only way to go. Why can't we just start labeling the conventional "poisoned" produce and make *them* pay additional costs to be certified, instead of the other way around?

As it is, the word *organic* can now only be legally used on products that are certified by one of several certifying organizations. The green-circled USDA Organic symbol has made it easily recognizable for consumers and has become the trusted symbol to look for when choosing organic foods. In the United States, certification is administered by the National Organic Program (NOP) of the USDA, which enforces organic product standards required by the Organic Food Production Act of 1990, and has the green-circle seal. Several other organizations certify products as well.

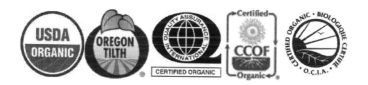

Multiple studies over the years have shown the difference in mineral content of organic versus conventional produce, and the general decline in nutrients over the last century. The differences are going to vary vastly based on what kind of soil the produce was grown in. A study from Rutgers University showed that mineral content varied radically in vegetables tested across the US. Tomatoes had anywhere from 1 to 1,938 ppm (dry matter) of iron, spinach had 1 to 117 ppm of manganese, and some lettuces had 4.5 times the amount of calcium.[16] This wasn't purely an organic versus conventional study, but one that verifies that what's in the soil is what goes into the produce. Then, what's in the produce goes in you!

Organic farming practices more often include compost and natural fertilizers that provide more nutrients to soil, which in turn is converted by the plant into nutrients that your body can absorb and use to help your body thrive. This is where knowing your farmer and buying organic and local can be of great value. If you know you're buying produce that has had excellent soil enrichment procedures in place, then you're going to get more nutrition from that vegetable or fruit while avoiding chemicals.

Another study, from 2014, found that organic produce had 17% higher amounts of overall phytonutrients that act as antioxidants and fight cell damage. Flavanones in particular were 69% higher. They were also lower in toxic cadmium.[17] Another study showed that organically raised chicken showed a significantly higher level of the good omega-3 fat in it versus conventional chicken.[18] You're also avoiding the chemicals that come in their feed. Organic is always a *better* choice, even though we'd much rather have pasture-raised chicken with even higher nutrient content.

Patients will often ask me, "How do you know that what you're buying that says it's organic is actually organic or any better for you?" In general, your odds of getting better nutrition and avoiding chemical residues are significantly higher when buying most things labeled as certified organic. Life has no guarantees, but, again, organic is always a *better* bet.

GMOS

This is a term that means Genetically Modified Organisms, and it has recently become much more recognized or mainstream. The World Health Organization (WHO) defines them as "Organisms, in which the genetic material (DNA) has been altered in a way that does not occur naturally.... It allows selected individual genes to be transferred from one organism into another, also between nonrelated species."[19] I'm sorry, did you just say altered DNA transfer between **nonrelated** species? Are you crazy?

Among other things, genetic engineering is used to give food traits that make its production more cost-efficient. GMO ingredients are showing up in more and more foods and products in the last ten years, and the amounts of them in our food supply continue to grow at an alarming rate. After the discovery of DNA in 1953, scientists began toying with this genetic material and realized that they could manipulate it to suit whatever particular need they had, without regard for safety of human consumption. Mixing the DNA of vegetables with e.coli bacteria? Talk about "mad scientists"!

By the early 1980s, the first GMO drugs began to emerge, and by the late '80s the first crops of corn, soy, tomatoes, and tobacco began to be farmed. In 1992, the United States FDA ruled that GMOs were "safe" and didn't require any special regulation. Oh good, I know I feel safe, don't you?

Since GMOs offered the ability to make foods more quickly, more insect-resistant, more cost-efficient, and more shelf-stable, how quickly do you think they began to spread among farmers, especially big farming operations? You guessed it…like wildfire! Why? What's the bottom line of all industry again? Money. Not that it's a bad thing to want to make a profit. Only, we need to do it without altering the Original Design for the foods that our bodies were designed to use.

I'm not really a conspiracy theory kind of guy. I'm not one to believe that there are evil puppet masters at the helm of big industry who'd like to kill you and your children. Rather, I believe they're regular people like you and me, who, since the '50s, have used technology and advancement in biochemistry to be more profitable so that they could take their kids on vacation and buy a new car. All the same things that motivate you and me to work every day have motivated people to make the food industry what it is today.

The challenge is, of course, that they've allowed the desire to make their industry more profitable to override the safety and health value of the foods that you and I consume. Inadvertently, they've created "fake foods" that are increasing their children's and now great-grandchildren's risk for everything from allergies and autoimmune disease to cancer.

At this point, researchers are uncertain of how many pure strains of non-GMO crops still remain, being that the issue of cross-pollination has become so widespread and problematic. What if you plant a field of GMO corn next to a field of non-GMO, or what some people call heirloom varieties of corn? You'll get some of the genetic material mixed and eventually be incapable of separating the two effectively. Unless we can get things drastically turned around in the US, it may only be in continental separation that there is hope.

As of the publication of this book, at least 26 countries have already banned GMOs, including Australia, India, China, France, Germany, Mexico, and Russia.[20] Why is the U.S. still producing and consuming GMOs? Sadly, it seems that money is all that matters to some.

The whole subject of GMOs goes right to the core of this book. I'll say it again, and I won't stop saying it: When we alter anything from the Original Design, we begin to have problems that can spiral out of control. With GMOs, we are disrupting and reengineering the very fabric of specifically designed DNA molecules, which are the blueprints for all living things. Have food engineers lost their minds? Who do they think they are? They're playing God. That usually doesn't turn out so well…for anyone.

When we try to find a cheaper, quicker, easier way, and change what God originally designed, we're going to pay for it dearly with our health. Haven't you found in your life that when you try to cut corners to help one aspect of whatever it is that you're doing, it ends up affecting another area or the entire endeavor as a whole? We know better than that.

The problem is, though, that no one in the food industry is going to admit to wrongdoing, whether it was intentional or not. The tobacco industry didn't volunteer guilt or "turn themselves in" when research made it clear that smoking was killing people by the millions. They were forced, by judges, after years of long court battles, to admit fault, pay fines, change labeling, and make people aware of the dangers of smoking. Yet cigarettes are still the number-one cause of "preventable" death today, meaning that a person chooses to smoke.

How hard do you think it'll be to get makers of corn puffs and wheaty O's to say, "Okay, you're right, we helped cause the number of cases of food allergies, inflammatory bowel disease, behavioral disorders, autoimmune disease, obesity, cardiovascular disease, and cancer to increase dramatically due to our use of chemicals, harsh processing and production of GMO foods. We're going to immediately switch to a locally based, non-GMO, organic farming model and we deeply apologize for the mess we created"? Not likely. Not on their own anyway.

There's too much money at stake and too much that's already in place. There's even more being planned for the future to continue "revolutionizing" how we produce food products in the US and around the world. GMO salmon already have preliminary FDA approval without any long-term studies on safety. They're not even required to. Brilliant.

"What can I do?" you ask. The only way to make big change is to "hit 'em where it counts" (aka the pocketbook). If we stop buying GMO, nonorganic or "conventional" items, we'll cause a dramatic shift in what is produced. We have to demand better. Seriously, the massive machines of industry don't give a flip what they're selling as long as you'll buy it and they make lots of money. If the public demands "poop on a stick," the industry doesn't care...they'll be happy to package it for you in different shapes, sizes, colors, and flavors to accommodate every desire. They simply want sales.

Let's give them sales, but let's demand high quality, unprocessed, organic, wild-caught (in the case of fish), pasture-raised (in the case of chicken and beef), non-GMO "real" food, instead of the engineered junk that's being cheaply made, sold at huge profits and destroying our health. Massive movements and sweeping changes always begin with the actions of a few. What you and I *buy* will drive the industry.

HOW MUCH AND EXACTLY WHAT SHOULD I EAT?

This is a question that I only get about 20 times a day, every day, from patients in my practice. This, of course, is the hardest question for any doctor or nutritionist to answer. The solution is quite a bit simpler than what it feels like or what you read in all of the conflicting ideas and reports out there.

Have you ever noticed that nearly every "reputable" source on the subject will quote studies that back up what they are saying? The sad answer is that you can find studies that support whatever you believe and choose to omit or ignore the studies that contradict what you believe. In my opinion, the simple fact is that no single diet plan will ever fit the needs of *every* person. How could it? You're an original. What you need is unique to you. Doesn't that make sense?

One of the principles that separates the idea of *The Original Design Diet* from other diets is that you are uniquely designed. To expect that someone else is going to know what kind of diet you need is ridiculous. The concept of Original Design creates a big problem for companies who want to create the next big diet craze. You can't package this "diet" and sell it to millions of people and have it be proprietary, because the basic premise is that an ideal diet is different for each individual. There are a few basic guidelines, though.

In general, all land animal products like beef, goat, or wild game should be pasture-raised or grass-fed in their natural, organic, chemical-free environments. This includes their dairy products as well, which should also be raw or unpasteurized, and not homogenized if at all possible…fresh from the farm. In order to properly digest these products, you need the enzymes that are active and naturally occurring in them, as well as other nutrients, before they are destroyed by the high heat of pasteurization.

All fish and seafood should be wild-caught in clean waters and fresh if possible. Fresh frozen is a good close second. Avoid farm-raised fish like the plague. They're cheaper for a reason, remember? You don't need GMO by-products or chemical residues—yuck. All birds like chicken, turkey, duck, and quail should also either be pasture-raised or wild—the same principle as the fish and land animals. They need to be eating the food in nature that they were designed to eat so that you can get the nutrients that you need.

All grains should be organically grown and, whenever possible, should be eaten sprouted. Don't freak out; you can buy organic sprouted-grain bread at most grocery stores now. Make sure all of your corn and rice products are organic too, or at least non-GMO. Nuts and seeds also need to be organic, and some people will do better with them slow-roasted at low temperatures. Look up "crispy nuts" on the Internet to find out more information.

All produce, like vegetables and fruit, should be organic and therefore, non-GMO. Produce, like berries, where you eat the outer surface that is sprayed is the most important to buy organic, but try to even get apples, oranges, and bananas organic too if you can. You help yourself, workers in the fields, and the environment when you buy organic. You also get better nutrient content and avoid the chemical pesticides and herbicides linked to all kinds of health problems, like allergies and infertility—even cancer. Luckily, there isn't much GMO produce out yet, but it's a-comin'.

Those are the basics. But based on your genetics, sex, age, body size, activity level, health level, time of year, and a number of other factors, you may need to eat something very different from other people. You may even need a different diet than close relatives, like siblings or parents. There are a few diets that make distinctions between individuals like the *Eat Right for Your Blood Type* diet, but I've had patients who followed "the rules" of some particular diet plan they read about in a book and did horribly, while others they knew did great. The Original Design Diet is the way to go!

Your body will tell you as you go along what's right for *you* in reference to how much fat, carbs, or protein you should eat and how it makes you feel. Most of you already know certain foods that you can't eat and foods that you have to eat to feel normal, regardless of what the book you read told you. One of the biggest issues is getting rid of the junk foods that are engineered and are really just a product of an industry after your money. Usually, they have very little *real* nutrition in them. When people stick to organic, unprocessed whole foods, they typically do really well.

Some will eat more protein from meat, and some will eat less. Some will eat more carbs; some will eat less, and so on. You'll learn what works best for you depending on how much you work out, your genetics, age, lifestyle, and how it makes you feel. Figuring it all out is part of the journey, and again, it's unique to *your* Original Design.

There's so much more critical information that I wanted to share with you in great detail about diet and nutrition. There is so much, in fact, that my awesome publisher realized that it was too much for one book and I had to cut out over 30,000 words from this chapter alone. All of that info and more fills an entire other book, my next book, *The Original Design Diet*. I can't wait to share it with you (we'll even have a cookbook, full of great recipes to go along with it). In the meantime, you've got a huge head start in understanding the important core principles of eating according to the Original Design. It's really simple.

The purpose of *this* book is to get you to see that it's the balance of *all* the pillars of health that is critically important to understand as the foundation for creating vibrant, complete health. Don't worry—I'll give you all the details you could ever want about diet and nutrition in *The Original Design Diet*. For now, however, start with the basics: Cut out the junk food and in moderation, enjoy the foods that were originally designed for you to eat. Your health will positively flourish!

CHAPTER 12

SUPPLEMENTS

As reported by the Centers for Disease Control and Prevention, more than half of Americans take supplements.[1] That statistic refers to vitamins, minerals, herbs, homeopathic remedies, fish oil, or anything in a bottle that is considered supplemental to the food that you eat. This is clearly a topic that is of a growing interest to most people in the modern world. The supplement industry "topped $32 billion in sales in 2012 and is projected to reach $60 billion by 2021."[2]

We're living in a time where people are getting sicker and sicker, but they're realizing it and they're looking for ways to improve their health. The only problem is that most people don't want to change their diet and lifestyle; they want a pill that will magically make them healthy while they eat pizza as they sit on the couch watching TV. It's funny, because when I ask patients if they *really* believe that they're going to find that "magic pill" that makes them look like a fitness magazine cover model without changing their diet and adding exercise, they all laugh and say, "Of course not."

Yet the diet pills, liquid potions, chemical-laden creams, and the fad supplements that promise major weight loss, ripped abs, big muscles, perfect skin, and the "fountain of youth" are selling like hotcakes! (Speaking of which, perhaps they should just eat less hotcakes.)

Something to note about supplements is that, contrary to what some people believe, supplements are not regulated or tested by the FDA in the same way as prescription and nonprescription drugs. They are considered under the category of "food" and thus are considered safe until proven unsafe according to the Dietary Supplement Health and Education Act.

Sadly, that means that you and I have no idea what's actually in a bottle of supplements when we purchase it. And we certainly don't know the quality of the ingredients in the final product either. We have to take the word of the manufacturer, who benefits financially from us buying their product. Hmmm.

Don't get me wrong here. I'm not looking for the federal government to begin restrictive regulations on supplements and to tell me what I can and can't buy. I'm never in favor of government intrusion. It just says to me that we, as consumers, need to know what we're buying and be sure that it's from a reputable company that's open and honest about where they source the ingredients for their products. They often get their raw products from the cheapest supplier in a distant land and put in useless fillers and harmful chemical additives.

WHERE DO VITAMINS COME FROM?

Vitamins weren't even discussed until they were discovered and named in 1912 by Polish-American biochemist Casimir Funk to describe an "amine" (chemical compound containing nitrogen) that was essential or "vital" to life, thus the term "vital amine" or vitamin. He realized that there was more to food than just fat, protein, carbohydrates, and minerals. At this point, he and others did a great deal of research connecting many diseases to vitamin deficiency. He even coproduced the first cod liver oil vitamin concentrate.[3] Shortly thereafter, the race was on by manufacturers to produce vitamins for mass consumption.

The problem was, how do you create large amounts of vitamins cheaply (for high profits) and make them shelf-stable? If you just stick fresh whole foods that are rich in certain vitamins in a bottle, they would spoil quickly, look gross, and taste even worse. Science was able to quickly come up with a "solution" to isolate nearly all of the known vitamins at the time and make them in one of two ways: crystalline vitamins or synthetic vitamins.

One way was to start with a real food, but then process it to isolate the vitamin through the use of high heat, chemicals, and solvents, which would distill out a pure, sterile (dead) crystalline powder (crystalline vitamins). The other way was to combine chemicals in a laboratory extracted from various other nonfood sources like coal tar and reconstruct synthetic compounds (synthetic vitamins) that looked just like the crystalline form. Unfortunately, most of the supplements on the market today are one of these two forms, and in my opinion they are nearly complete junk. They likely create more harm than good.

The medical profession is famous for telling patients that they're wasting time and money on bottled "vitamins" and that all they're really getting is "expensive urine." Guess what? For the most part, I think they're absolutely right. Many of the supplements on the market may not even have in them what they say they do because they're not held accountable for what's inside the bottle until they are "proven" otherwise.

The attorney general of the state of New York recently published results of commissioned tests on some popular herbal supplements available in national chains like GNC, Walgreens, Target, and Walmart. After testing hundreds of bottles, they found that four out of five did not even contain the herbs that were listed on the label.[4] While the type of analysis that was used, which is called the DNA barcoding technique, is somewhat controversial, these types of studies have been done before, using different methods and have come up with similar results. It just highlights a good point.

So, let me stress this again: You need to know your supplement company and be confident in them and what they produce. Where they source materials from to make their products and what their standards are is extremely important to know and understand. Don't just take the word of the person who "told you so" at a sales meeting or the kid working at the vitamin store. Do a little of your own research. You're about to put these pills in your body after purchasing them with your hard-earned money. They should be high quality.

WHAT'S IN THERE?

Again, a major issue with most supplements is that the "vitamins" themselves are a cheap, man-made, synthetic form of their naturally occurring, living counterparts that were originally designed to exist in real food and to nourish your body. It's often hard to even trust "research" quoted by manufacturers.

One study, reported on March 26, 1999 by Reuters, found that women whose diets were high in vitamin E (an antioxidant) showed a reduction in LDL ("bad" cholesterol) oxidation, or plaque build-up on artery walls. This is great, right? Vitamin E helps protect against cardiovascular disease. Yee-haw! Soon thereafter, there was a mad dash from vitamin companies to mass produce and sell synthetic vitamin E by pushing it with the claim that "research shows" that their product is heart healthy. Umm, not really.

You see, there's just one little problem. What the study *actually* said is that the women whose "diets" (meaning the food that they actually ate) that were naturally high in vitamin E gave them the added health benefit. It said nothing about them benefitting from synthetic vitamin E supplements.

In fact, it was stated by the lead researcher of the study that the synthetic form of vitamin E, (DL-)alpha-tocopherol, is what is commonly found in vitamin E supplements, but it's the naturally occurring form that's protective. It's amazing how easily we trust that what was found in research is actually what is being offered to us in a bottle. The synthetic forms are not only of little value to the body, but they may actually harm the body. In her presentation, she also said of the test subjects that "the more (synthetic) vitamin E they took, the worse their LDL oxidation (cardiovascular disease risk)." Oops!

Unfortunately, that's not the only issue. She also stated that the synthetic form displaces the natural form in our tissues, so that now "all you've got" is the synthetic form instead of the naturally occurring form that's in our food.[5] This is something that I call competitive inhibition.

What this basically means is that when both the naturally occurring form and the synthetic form of a vitamin is present in the digestive tract at the same time, the synthetic vitamin disrupts the natural form from being absorbed efficiently and used effectively in the body. Not only does the synthetic form potentially not even help you, but it could actually hurt you by blocking your body from absorbing and using some of the naturally occurring vitamins in the foods that you eat.

Have you ever had a key on your keychain that looked so similar to another key that, occasionally, you'd mistakenly put it in the keyhole that was designed for the other key? Now imagine a long hallway with thousands of doors and keyholes in each of the doorknobs. Let's say you went along that hallway and inserted the wrong key into each keyhole. The keys fit, but didn't turn the locks, and so you broke them off in the keyholes while trying to make them work. Now I come along with the correct key for each lock, but there's already a key in the keyhole, blocking my correct key from going in the lock and unlocking the door.

Many synthetic "vitamins" don't even occur in nature, and the ones that do are still pathetic rip-offs of their naturally occurring counterparts.

Your gastrointestinal system, namely the small intestine, works much the same way in that it has thousands of receptor sites designed for specific nutrients to be absorbed into the bloodstream and used in the body. However, when taking a synthetic supplement, we may "clog up" that beautifully designed system with a man-made chemical that looks close to the real thing, but won't function correctly. This could potentially create absolute chaos and illness or disease that affects you now and for the rest of your life.

Recently, the National Institutes of Health reported that "synthetically produced alpha-tocopherol…is only half as active as the same amount of the natural form. People need approximately 50% more IU of synthetic alpha tocopherol from dietary supplements and fortified foods to obtain the same amount of the nutrient as from the natural form."

They went on to say, "Research has not found any adverse effects from consuming vitamin E in food. However, high doses of alpha-tocopherol *supplements* can cause hemorrhage," increase "the risk of cataract formation," and "results from the recently published, large SELECT trial show that vitamin E supplements (400 IU/day) may harm adult men in the general population by increasing their risk of prostate cancer."[6]

Many synthetic "vitamins" don't even occur in nature, and the ones that do are still pathetic rip-offs of their naturally occurring counterparts. We need vitamins in the form we were designed to get them—in their originally designed form, which is the third and correct form.

Naturally occurring vitamins are "alive" and often referred to as "vitamin complexes" that contain the central vitamin with many additional enzymes, coenzymes, and cofactors. They surround it and cause the whole complex to become readily absorbable and highly active or effective in the body. In a naturally occurring whole-food vitamin, the only thing that's removed from the food source is the moisture and some fiber. The chart below is a comparison of naturally occurring vitamins and their dietary sources versus the synthetically produced versions of the same vitamin and what they're derived from.

Vitamin	Top Food Sources	Common Synthetic Name on Labels[7]	Synthetic Source, Chemicals Used in Processing, and Fun Facts
Vitamin A	Sweet potatoes, carrots, spinach, kale, greens, romaine lettuce, cantaloupe, peppers, broccoli	Vitamin A acetate, retinal or vitamin A palmitate, beta-carotene	Refined oils, methanol, petroleum esters, acetylene, and benzene, which causes leukemia in humans. Nice.
Vitamin B-1	Asparagus, sunflower seeds, peas, flax, Brussels sprouts, spinach, cabbage, romaine lettuce	Thiamin mononitrate, thiamin hydrochloride, thiamin HCL	Coal tar derivatives, hydrochloric acid and ammonia with acetonitrile, which can cause respiratory failure. Good idea.
Vitamin B-2	Spinach, most greens, eggs, asparagus, milk, broccoli, mushrooms, green beans, kale	Riboflavin	Synthetically produced with 2N acetic acid…requires using gloves, goggles, and safety devices. Fun!
Vitamin B-3	Tuna, chicken, turkey, salmon, lamb, beef, sardines, peanuts, shrimp, sweet potatoes, brown rice	Niacin, niacinamide	Coal tar derivative, 3-cyanopyridine, acid and ammonia…wait, isn't that in fertilizer and floor cleaner? Cool.
Vitamin B-5	Mushrooms, avocado, sweet potatoes, lentils, chicken, peas, turkey, broccoli, salmon, beef	Panthenol, pantothenic acid, calcium pantothenate	Isobutyraldehyde condensed with formaldehyde: you know…the stuff used to store dead science specimens. Yum.
Vitamin B-6	Tuna, turkey, beef, chicken, salmon, sweet potatoes, spinach, sunflower seeds, bananas, beans	Pyridoxine HCL, pyridoxine hydrochloride	Petroleum ester and hydrochloric acid with formaldehyde, which is great for making car parts…not body parts.
Vitamin B-7	Peanuts, almonds, eggs, sweet potatoes, oats, salmon, walnuts, tomatoes, onions, carrots, milk	Biotin	Chemically produced in a lab using fumaric acid created by oxidation of benzene or butane. Sounds natural.
Vitamin B-9	Lentils, asparagus, spinach, beans, broccoli, greens, Brussels sprouts, romaine lettuce, nuts	Folic acid, folate	Processed from petroleum derivatives, acids, and acetylene…as in blow torch fuel. Awesome!
Vitamin B-12	Sardines, salmon, tuna, cod, lamb, scallops, shrimp, beef, milk, eggs, turkey, chicken	Cyanocobalamin, hydroxycobalamin	Made from cobalamins reacted with cyanide…yep, cyanide…the poison. Enjoy that.

(continued)

Vitamin	Top Food Sources	Common Synthetic Name on Labels[7]	Synthetic Source, Chemicals Used in Processing, and Fun Facts
Vitamin C	Papaya, bell peppers, broccoli, Brussels sprouts, strawberries, pineapples, oranges, kiwi, kale	Ascorbic acid, sodium ascorbate, other mineral ascorbates, pycnogenols	GMO corn sugar hydrogenated with acetone... the flammable liquid used in nail polish remover. Yay!
Vitamin D	Cod liver oil, other marine oils, salmon, swordfish, tuna, trout, sardines, milk, eggs, (sunlight)	Cholecalciferol, D1, D2, D3 (isolated), D4, ergosterol, lumisterol	Solvent extracted or from irradiated animal fat, cattle brains, or sheep skin secretions. Sounds delicious.
Vitamin E	Wheat germ oil, sunflower seeds, almonds, hazelnuts, spinach, peanuts, shrimp	All vitamin E acetates, mixed tocopherols, d or dL-alpha-tocopherol	Refined oils, trimethylhydroquinone and isophytol also used in toilet cleaners and detergents. Perfect!
Vitamin K	Kale, spinach, greens, parsley, broccoli, Brussels sprouts, basil, romaine lettuce, asparagus, cabbage	Vitamin K3, menadione, phytonadione, dihydro-vitamin K1, naphthoquinone	Coal tar derivative produced with p-allelic-nickel...all good for making coins...not something going in my body.

HOW MUCH DO I NEED TO TAKE?

An important factor to consider when it comes to supplementation is the dosage or how much you should take and how often. As we all know, supplements aren't cheap. If we're going to spend our hard-earned money on a bottle of something, not only do we want to know what's in there but we need to know how much of it to take.

It requires a certain amount of the active compounds of a particular nutrient to get a desired response. By that I mean that unless you get an appropriate dose of a vitamin or herb, it may not benefit you enough to even notice. You may then make an incorrect assumption that what you took isn't working. It would be like licking a Tylenol when you've got a splitting headache and then wondering why it didn't help with the pain. You might even go so far as to tell a friend, "You know, Tylenol has never helped me with headaches, and I'm not sure it even works."

Thousands of people have taken a supplement that had little of the active ingredient in it, or they simply took an inappropriately small dosage, but either way they decided that it didn't work for them. This is where the guidance of a trained food-sourced nutritionist can really make a big difference in the effectiveness of your supplementation. If you're going it alone, the recommendations on the bottle are generally safe but not necessarily representative of what you may need.

To aggressively treat a condition that you're experiencing, a nutritionist might have you double or triple the amount that you might normally take for a short period of time in order to build up your system and help normalize function or boost tissue repair. Based on your weight, age, or particular health issues, you might need a different dosage as well. Most dosages on bottles will be based on the weight of an average adult. If we take the average weight of men at 196 and women at 166, that averages to 181.[8] Therefore, if an adult dosage of a food-based supplement is two capsules per meal, then it would make sense that a child that weighs ninety pounds might take one capsule per meal.

One other thing I also consistently tell patients is to take their supplements in smaller amounts, multiple times throughout the day, instead of all at once. Instead of taking six capsules of something in the morning, I suggest taking two capsules three times per day (with meals and plenty of water). This just makes sense.

For instance, while you may need 80 ounces of water throughout the day, you can't possibly drink and use 80 ounces of water in the first ten minutes of the day. You also wouldn't eat all three meals of the day, and snacks, for breakfast, would you? It's just more than your body can process at one time. In the same way, it's best to spread your supplements out throughout the day so that they can be at high levels in your bloodstream all day long. This makes them much more effective and available when needed.

HOW LONG DO I TAKE THEM?

Some people might take the time to choose a good supplement and take the appropriate dosage but then stop short of the appropriate length of treatment that's needed to get the desired effect. Several months might have been needed for it to sufficiently accumulate in their systems to have made the intended change, but they only took it for two weeks. This would be like having a severe, life-threatening bacterial infection and only taking the antibiotic your MD prescribed for one or two days, when it was suggested to take it for ten days. It may have little effect on the condition. Again, this is where working with a trained professional in nutrition will give you the best chance at being helped with your particular condition by giving you a good quality supplement, in the right amount, over the correct period of time.

When I think about how long a person should take a particular supplement, I often equate it to the analogy of a starving child in a third-world country. It brings to mind images of this little person with a distended abdomen and cracked lips and various other health issues. Whenever I see these pictures or videos, they break my heart and usually bring tears to my eyes. It's easy to imagine that this child is going to need more than one healthy meal. In fact, it's not going to be over the course of a few days or weeks, but typically many months and sometimes years before that little body is sufficiently nourished and restored back to health.

Like that starving child, our bodies repair in much the same way. We're typically not in a severe state of starvation, disease, or dysfunction. However, some people have been eating quite poorly for a long time. For them, it will take many months or years to undo the damage and restore the tissues to their normal function…back to their Original Design.

On a personal note, my wife and I sponsor several children on different continents to at least do a small part to change that situation. We also support several ministries and charities that provide worldwide relief. If we all make a small sacrifice to help, then together, we can stop world hunger.

Research shows that replacing different cells takes different periods of time in the body. The lining of your intestines could be replaced in as quickly as five days, whereas the liver could take about a year. While some of our brain cells are replaced frequently, others are with us for our entire lives and are never replaced.[9] Since many tissues and organs will need a great deal of time to improve, be patient…time is your friend.

Natural alternatives can potentially work just as good as or better than the drugs used for the same condition.

WHEN TO SUPPLEMENT

There are several factors to consider when deciding whether or not to take a supplement. Did I mention that you'll benefit from working with a trained and experienced food-based nutritionist? ☺ However, your own personal research is always of tremendous value too. There are many resources in bookstores and online to help you figure out what issues you might be experiencing and what supplements could help alleviate them. There are some common scenarios, though, that often benefit from supplementation. Here are a few.

If you travel a great deal for work, then it's likely that you'll find it difficult to find any organic produce or "clean" meats as described in the previous chapter. You're often presented with few options of what to eat and so adding supplements to your diet will significantly help round out your nutritional needs.

People who live in rural areas where the produce section in the local grocery store consists of wilted lettuce and a few mealy tomatoes with bugs flying around them are gonna need some serious help. Hopefully, though, you can grow some of your own veggies. It's fun, tasty, and extremely nutritious as you can control how they're grown.

Those in poor health, who've been diagnosed with a particular condition but who choose not to take potentially dangerous medications could be great candidates for supplementation. Specifically supporting certain organs or systems in your body can help get you back on track. Other issues in your health might clear up as well, since everything is so interconnected. Natural alternatives can potentially work just as good as or better than the drugs used for the same condition. Listen to me very carefully though: **Always** check with your doctor before stopping any medication. Stopping a medication all at once can have really devastating consequences.

Nursing mothers are another group who not only need to nourish themselves but want to ensure that their milk is of the highest nutrient content for their baby. What the mom eats has a definite influence on what's in her milk. However, it's amazing to me how her milk may be in pretty good shape, as it'll get many of the needed nutrients from her own body (organs, bones, fat, muscle) if she's been eating poorly. Regardless, we want to make sure that if her diet is lacking, we add some core supplements to supply what's missing. Once babies are weaned off of breast milk, their nutrient intake becomes directly related to what they eat.

Little kids are at risk of nutritional deficiencies, as many of them can be picky eaters. Sadly, many parents will cater to this pickiness and give their children engineered foods that have little nutritional value and may even cause significant harm. To name just a few: allergies, learning disabilities, behavioral challenges, susceptibility to getting sick, and diseases like diabetes and obesity in kids have been linked to poor eating habits. Have you ever heard a parent say, "Little Jimmy just won't eat anything but mac'n cheese or bread"? Umm, well, we need to have a talk. That's not all Jimmy's fault.

The elderly are also a classic group of people who greatly benefit from nutritional supplementation, because they often severely limit their food choices as cooking becomes a big chore. Also, convenience foods that are chosen for ease of access are nearly always lacking in nutrition.

I remember going to a friend's grandparents' house and seeing them on their recliners with a small table of "cookie jars" between them filled with crackers, chips, cookies, pretzels, and popcorn. Right next to the jars were about 20 different Rx medications for everything from diabetes to cholesterol and blood pressure meds. Think there might be any connection there?

One critical thing to consider here is that as we age, we digest and absorb less and less of what's in our food. This is a big problem. Certain research suggests that the elderly may only get about half the amount of nutrients from the same foods eaten by someone half their age. A nutritional epidemiologist who spoke at the Institute of Medicine's Food Forum explained how "recent research demonstrates that because older adults' abilities to absorb and utilize many nutrients become less efficient, their nutrient requirements actually increase."[10]

This would imply that when we get older, we get less than what we need, even if we eat well. Since it's probably part of the Original Design to need less nutrients as we age, we don't have to get too worried or go overboard on supplements. We just need to be smart, at any age, and ensure that we're getting what we need overall.

YOU'RE READY

Now that you've had a short course in supplementation, you'll be much better equipped to look at and analyze all of the bottles on your shelves, and the ones at the stores. Very well-meaning people have tried and will continue to try to sell you supplements that are cheaply made and add little value to your body. Some could possibly even create harm. Most of their motivation for getting you to buy their supplements is to create income for themselves, not to make you healthy.

Use your newfound understanding of what's in supplements to evaluate any that are recommended to you, even if by a professional. Knowledge is power. Use it to your advantage and stop wasting money on junky "chemical pills" that are cheap counterfeits of the real thing. Take an honest look at your diet and only use supplementation as a way to fill in the gaps.

As I've said, we were designed to get all the nutrients that we need from the foods that are on this earth. The nutrients of these *real foods* (not synthetic chemicals) were also designed to be easily assimilated in our bodies and used as the fuel to keep us extremely healthy. However, the truth is that in this day and age of eating out and living on processed junk food, probably all of us fall short of getting everything we need from our diet, even if we try hard. For this reason, supplementation is important.

For me and my family, though, supplementation is more important during travel, times of illness, for a specific need, or due to childhood dietary pickiness. If you're having some health issues that you suspect may be due to improper eating and/or a lack of certain nutrients, then—you guessed it—I highly suggest connecting with a well-trained nutritionist who understands whole-food nutrition.

If you simply rely on information that you've received from friends and family, or articles that you've read or things that you've heard, it's going to be an extremely frustrating exercise to choose appropriate supplements. Commonly, most people go online or to a health-food store, supplement store, or even the vitamin aisle at the grocery store, and pick something at random. They'll choose based on an advertisement that they've heard, the packaging, or the perceived value due to the size and cost of the bottle: "Hey Ma, look at this here bottle, it's huge and dirt cheap!"

As you might imagine, those are really poor ways of choosing which supplement you need. Just because a large bottle at a low-cost seems like a good value doesn't mean that you're getting a good product that'll benefit you. Advertisers aren't dumb. They've studied human nature and they're going to make their product as appealing as possible. Don't get duped!

Again, you need to be familiar with the company and how they source their raw products to make their final products. There are a few supplement companies in the resource section of this book who have proven track records and have data to back up their claims of potency and content. If you need to support your diet with a supplement for any number of reasons, I strongly urge you to choose a good supplement company and a good nutritionist. Either with help or on your own, you can now choose more wisely and feel more confident that you're getting something in a capsule that's as close as possible to the Original Design for your health.

PILLAR IV

SPIRITUAL

CHAPTER 13

INTELLIGENT DESIGN

Intelligent Design (ID) is defined by Webster's dictionary as the claim that "certain features of the universe and of living things are best explained by an intelligent cause, not an undirected process...." I would be remiss if I didn't discuss ID in this book, as it has some obvious parallels to the Original Design. Learning about ID helps us understand that we and every living thing on our planet are not just a random accident, but are intentionally designed.

There is a specific design to every intricate detail of our bodies. Really understanding how that design works helps us see how all the pillars of health were intelligently designed to fit together to create the Original Design for health. It also helps us come to a place that solidifies our faith and belief in God, who is the Designer.

While I won't cover everything about ID, I do believe it's important to get a solid, basic understanding of this subject when talking about our overall health. I'll give links to other organization's websites, under the Resources section if you want to learn more. The basic outline and much of this chapter comes from the amazing, eye-opening DVD entitled *Unlocking the Mystery of Life* by Illustra Media. It's incredibly well done and I highly recommend that you get it and show it to your entire family and friends if this information interests you.

WHERE DOES LIFE COME FROM?

The question of the origin of life has been pondered by the vast majority of humans on earth. We want to know because we want to know where *we* come from. We're going to jump into some information that is a little detailed and will remind you of biology class, but it helps set the stage for understanding just how unbelievably amazing our design is!

To explain the existence of life on earth, we first have to account for the origin of the essential building blocks for every living cell on earth, which are complex molecules called proteins. Even simple cells are made of thousands of kinds of proteins. The functions of proteins come from their highly complex and unique three-dimensional shapes. Proteins themselves are made up of smaller chemical components called amino acids that are linked together in long chains.

There's an incredible degree of detail in the architecture within protein-forming amino acids. In nature, 22 different types of amino acids are used to construct protein chains. Biologists compare them to the 26 letters of the alphabet. You can arrange the letters of the alphabet into an unbelievable number of possible combinations. However, it's the exact arrangement and grouping of those letters that determine whether you've made a sentence that you can understand, or just complete nonsense. Take a look at these two sentences: "ywIvhy eo loluitrtl mhe aa!" and "I love you with all my heart!" One is designed and the other is random. Can you tell which is which? Of course you can. I'm just being silly, but the fact that it's obvious is part of the point.

There are roughly 30,000 distinct types of proteins, each made up of a different combination of the exact same 22 amino acids. They are arranged into chains that can be hundreds of units long. If the amino acids are sequenced correctly, then the chain will fold into a functioning protein. It's that exact shape or architectural design of the protein that determines its function. If it's assembled with just one amino acid in the wrong sequence, then it'll be destroyed inside the cell because it's not functional.

The question is *what* produces this exact sequencing of amino acids to give rise to the proteins that combine to form the cell parts, then combine to form the cell, which then combines together with other cells to form tissues that form together to create organs, which come together to create a complete, fully functional human body? Since the sequencing is so critical to creating something that actually works, we have to find out how it "knows" how to connect together appropriately. Where does the set of instructions come from for even the smallest of molecules to correctly combine together? It's called DNA.

The amount of information in human DNA is roughly equivalent to 12 sets of encyclopedias, which equals 384 volumes worth of detailed information that would fill 48 feet of library shelves!

THE MIND-BLOWING DISCOVERY OF DNA

Proteins can't self-assemble without DNA—it's critical to their formation. As scientists began to decode the human DNA molecule, they found something they weren't expecting: an extremely highly detailed "language" composed of about three billion genetic letters. (A tad more complex than our simple language of 26 letters.) Unbelievable! "One of the most extraordinary discoveries of the twentieth century was that DNA actually stores information—the detailed instructions for assembling proteins—in the form of a four-character digital code."[1]

I know it's hard to wrap your head around, but think about this. The amount of information in human DNA is roughly equivalent to 12 sets of encyclopedias, which equals 384 volumes worth of detailed information that would fill 48 feet of library shelves! This is not random gobbledygook, but perfect intelligently designed plans for making proteins, all of which do something completely unique! Are you kidding me? Wow!

Scientists started looking at DNA with more and more detail as technology increased and better microscopes became available. Imagine them looking inside the DNA molecule, expecting to find some random goop, but instead they found 384 books worth of tiny detailed blueprints for every single part of our bodies. Amazing! Yet in their actual size, which is only two-millionths of a millimeter thick, a teaspoon of DNA, according to molecular biologist Michael Denton, could contain all the information needed to build the proteins for all the species of organisms that have ever lived on the earth, and "there would still be enough room left for all the information in every book ever written."[2] I don't know about you, but that just blows my mind! The chemical code in DNA is the most densely packed and elaborately detailed assembly of information in the entire universe.

Think about how impossibly unlikely this would be: Take the letters from several Scrabble board games and throw them up in the air. When they land, they not only have to land in several absolutely perfectly straight lines, but they have to spell out the Declaration of Independence without a *single* spelling or punctuation mistake. Now consider that the specific genetic instructions or DNA required to build the proteins in even the simplest of one-celled organisms would fill hundreds of pages of printed words, not just one. That is unfathomable!

DARWIN'S EXPLANATION

Darwinism is defined as the theory that species originate by evolving with variation, from a parent form, through the "natural selection" of the specific individuals that are best adapted for reproductive success. In other words, whether by random mutation or "luck of the draw," some creatures within a species are better able to survive and have babies with similarly "lucky" features, thereby slowly eliminating the "weak" and promoting the "strong." Darwin discussed this in the term that we've all heard, "survival of the fittest."

Interestingly, in his book, *On the Origin of Species*, Darwin himself said, "If it could be demonstrated that any complex organ existed which could not possibly have been formed by numerous successive, slight modifications, my theory would absolutely break down."[3] I've got news, Chuck.

Since the advent of the electron microscope, scientists have discovered many complex "organs" or parts of living organisms that can't be explained by natural selection, (e.g., the flagellar motor), and for several reasons. His theory *has* "absolutely broken down," as he put it. No disrespect to Darwin, he was a brilliant scientist, but it's true. If you want to get into this fascinating concept more, look up the term "irreducible complexity" on the internet.

Also, "natural selection" could not have functioned as a law of nature before the existence of the first living cell, because, by definition, it can only act upon organisms that are capable of *reproducing themselves*. Without DNA there are no cells, and without cells there is no self-replication, and without self-replication there is no "natural selection." This proves you can't use "natural selection" to explain the origin of DNA without assuming the existence of the very thing that you're trying to explain! Chance, natural selection, and self-organization all fail to explain the origin of the highly detailed genetic information in DNA. There is one alternative, however: Intelligent Design.

RECOGNIZING INTELLIGENCE

Since the time of Charles Darwin, scientists have accepted a convention or definition of science that excluded design as a scientific explanation. It's called methodological naturalism, which means that if you're going to be "scientific," you have to limit yourself to explanations that only have *natural* causes. You're not allowed to consider intelligence as a cause. Francis Crick,

Nobel laureate in DNA research, said, "Biologists must constantly keep in mind that what they see was not designed, but evolved."[4] Well, that's not scientific at all, that's philosophical!

Aren't scientists supposed to consider *all* of the options and *all* of the facts? Oh, and by the way, why would you constantly have to keep reminding yourself that it's *not* designed? It keeps coming to mind as the obvious answer, doesn't it? The truth is that we recognize intelligent design in things all the time. It's part of normal human reasoning to recognize the effects of intelligent design. Intelligence is about as natural as it gets.

Let's say you were to walk through the seemingly endless Egyptian desert and cross mile after mile of sandy, wind-swept terrain and then suddenly happen upon the pyramids. Eventually you even get close enough to see the hieroglyphics inscribed on their walls. Do you think that you'd you think to yourself, "Wow, what an amazing set of perfectly shaped and equal-sided random stone structures of magnificent scale! Clearly, the wind and rain must've accidently created them and miraculously etched what *appears* to be some form of writing and symbols into the walls…but that can't be. It must simply be a coincidence in its similarity to man-made buildings and ancient writing"? Oh, come on, of course you wouldn't. You and I both would instantly recognize them as Egyptian architecture and writing. At a bare minimum, we'd recognize them as having been designed by some intelligent being and not naturally occurring by chance.

Every day, scientists use common sense to differentiate between random, naturally occurring events and obviously intelligently designed ones.

In the news recently, there was an article about some archaeologists who discovered a massive circular pile of rocks located underwater in the

Sea of Galilee. They say it's definitely human-made and was probably built on land, only later to be covered by the Sea of Galilee as the water levels rose. "The shape and composition of the submerged structure does not resemble any *natural* feature. We therefore conclude that it is *man-made…*" the researchers wrote.[5] That's a perfect example of what I'm talking about.

This is the conclusion of educated *scientists*. This is not a guess by some random dudes who watch a lot of shows on the Discovery channel. Every day, scientists use common sense to differentiate between random, naturally occurring events and obviously intelligently designed ones. In science, we cannot lose sight of reality and common sense when trying to decipher the world around us.

How *do* we scientifically determine that something has been intelligently designed versus being designed by accident? It's simple. Humans notice improbably complex objects with recognizable patterns, also described as things of small probability and specific detail. Together, these two things are what scientists call "information."

For over 30 years, scientists at the Search for Extraterrestrial Intelligence Institute (SETI) have been scanning radio signals from space for a specific sequence of information-rich patterns that could be recognizable as intelligent. They look for complexity and pattern, not just a simple repeating signal or static. They're looking for that specific kind of "information" with small probability and specific detail. It's just like in the movie *Contact* that I mentioned earlier, where one of the lead characters, a scientist, is listening with headphones to "static" from outer space, hoping to find patterns—intelligently designed ones.

INFORMATION IS THE SCIENCE OF THE 21ST CENTURY

In the 19th century, scientists believed that all of science was based on two foundations: matter and energy. But now in the 21st century, we realize that there's a new, *third* factor that must be considered: information.

Bill Gates said in his 1995 book, *The Road Ahead*, that "DNA is like a computer program but far, far more advanced than any software ever created."[6] Designing software is not an accidental process and it's not simple; it's highly detailed with purpose. Bill doesn't use random number generators or wind and erosion and chance to create software programs. He hires the most intelligent software engineers he can find to *design* software for his company. Everything we know about information-rich systems tells us that it arises from intelligent design.

Likewise, *every* living cell of *every* living organism has highly detailed information in it that we call DNA. Where are we going to assume that it comes from? There are simply no natural causes that create information; only intelligent designers make meaningful information.

If we conclude that there *is* an intelligent designer who created DNA, then you can look into nature and expect to find order and beauty and design in all living things. What we see inside DNA and what we see in the world all around us can *only* be explained as a product of an intelligent designer who had an Original Design for all things.

ID'S EFFECT ON SPIRITUAL HEALTH

The scientists who formed the idea of ID don't necessarily like to draw conclusions openly about a connection to faith in God as it's not the main point of their theory. I, however, will draw that conclusion as I'm discussing it in *my* book. When we say that there's an intelligent design, it implies that there's a design*er*. In my opinion, that designer is God. The implications, then, are huge for our spiritual beliefs! In the end, if there is an intelligent design, and if there is a God or a Creator if you like, then you have to live your life differently in light of His existence.

Understanding the amazing complexity of DNA and the design of all living things, I can't help but realize that we are fearfully and wonderfully made. DNA is not an accident, and neither are we. Understanding *how* we're made helps strengthen the spiritual pillar of the foundation of health for all of us. In knowing that there is a design for even the smallest of molecules, it solidifies in my heart that there was and is a plan, or an Original Design, for everything, including little ole me. That knowledge nourishes my spiritual health and gives me a certainty that improves my overall health and happiness.

CHAPTER 14

FAITH

I'll be honest with you (don't worry, I was being honest before too; it's just a figure of speech): This was both the easiest and the toughest chapter for me to write. Everyone knows that when you go to meet your girlfriend's parents for the first time, or attend a dinner party with a diverse crowd, or hang around the water cooler at the office, there are two subjects you never discuss: religion and politics. Luckily, this book is no place to discuss politics. The other one, though—that other taboo subject—is, of course, the very personal, polarizing, hot, and controversial subject of faith.

HOW FAITH STRENGTHENS YOUR HEALTH

We all have what C. S. Lewis called "inconsolable longings" that nothing in this world can satisfy. Nothing. No matter what we try, *only* a relationship with God and His love will ever fill that void. We have a deep desire to know if there is a God, where we came from, if we'll ever find someone to love, if someone will ever love us in return, and to know where we're going when our time on earth is done. These spiritual questions aren't light subjects; they have deep meaning and implications for how we think, feel, function, and live our lives. And they greatly affect our overall health and happiness.

Our core beliefs serve as "internal navigators" that guide us through all the ups and downs of life. Our faith is a foundational part of our core beliefs. What we believe determines much of how we value and take care of ourselves. If we have the faith to believe that we were specifically and purposefully designed, then we think differently, act differently, and naturally take better care of ourselves.

As there are millions of books written about faith, I'll leave it to those experts and your specific needs to guide you to the appropriate information. However, there are a number of things that I find interesting and important as it relates to the connection between faith and health that I want to share.

One critical idea tying spiritual health to your overall health is the idea of connecting with *the* Source and Designer of all things—God. Just like our cell phones need to plug into a power source and recharge, so do we. God is our constant source of power that will never waiver. We've got to connect with Him daily to renew and restore our energy reserves and to be able to handle what comes our way each and every day. Some of the following ideas have helped my faith, and I hope to help you solidify your own faith and how important it is to the spiritual pillar of your foundation of health.

Just like our cell phones need to plug into a power source and recharge, so do we.

A FOUNDATIONAL TRUTH

Whether at the desk in my study, hiking in the mountains, or sitting on a quiet stretch of pristine beach while pondering the writing of this book, I was frequently confronted with a real and unmistakable, impassable, and foundational truth. I have come to the conclusion that without faith in God, nothing in this world has a frame of reference, significance, or meaning. Why on earth would anyone care about optimal health, relationships, or future generations, if there's no purpose for humans to be on this whirling globe? It would all seem pretty meaningless.

For us to have true peace in our hearts, we need to understand that God is real, that He designed us, and that He loves us. This is so important. We have to accept His love in order for our lives to be established on a foundation of peace. The writer of Proverbs said, "A heart at peace gives life to the body..." (Proverbs 14:30 NIV). Otherwise, there is way too much uncertainty and instability. It was often reported that Charles Darwin suffered from severe anxiety. I can see why; sadly, he had no peace in his heart. When you believe that you're an accident and that life has no meaning, it's a sad, unsettling, scary, and unhealthy place to be.

We're told in public school that all we are is one big cosmic accident, and we began as clumps of elements that collected into microorganisms, which grew into worms, which accidently sprouted arms, climbed out onto the beach, and huddled in a cave for an extremely long time. Then we mutated into a monkey and threw a rock at something, thereby creating a spark that started a fire, and as the French would say, "Voilà!" we became modern man! I've gotta say...I'm a little skeptical of that explanation. I mean, really? I don't know about you, but it kinda seems like a stretch to me.

All kidding aside, and with all due respect to my fellow doctors and scientists, I firmly believe that it takes a significantly greater amount of *faith* to believe in a totally random kind of evolution than it does to believe in a loving, all-knowing, all-powerful God who designed us as humans, the earth, and everything in it for us to live on and enjoy. The idea of the "Big Bang" could be called "accidental perfection." It requires millions of leaps of faith for everything to have turned out as perfectly as it did versus just one leap of faith...the leap that says there is one God, one Designer who had one Original Design. One.

**"All of us believe something,
it's just a matter of *what* we believe."**

And, by the way, before my scientific friends get their shorts in a bunch, I'm not saying there's no such thing as "evolution" or adaptation. The previous chapter on ID puts the whole idea in a really good frame of reference. You'd have to be really uninformed or dogmatic to not recognize what we've discovered in science. There's clear evidence that's been documented over the last few centuries of how many species of animals and plants have adapted and "evolved" into different forms due to a multitude of environmental factors. Yet we're faced with the very real truth that the *most likely* scenario is that everything in this world and the processes that govern adaptation were originally designed by an intelligent force or...God.

The question is not *if* you're a "believer." The question is whether you believe that God created the earth and everything in it through some unknown timeline, or that you believe that there is no God and it all just happened completely randomly. All of us believe something, it's just a matter of *what* we believe. As for my personal faith as a Christian, I've been through many ups and downs, but I can say that I wholeheartedly believe in God, the Author of the Original Design. As I've stated, I believe that He created everything in the universe and that when I die I will go to heaven for eternity.

In the book based on a true story *Heaven Is for Real*, which was recently made into a movie, a four-year-old boy named Colton, who, during emergency surgery, slips out of consciousness and enters heaven. He survives and begins talking about being able to look down and see the doctor operating and his dad praying in the waiting room. The family didn't know what to believe but soon the evidence became clear.

While in heaven, Colton said he met his miscarried sister, whom no one had told him about, and his great-grandfather who died 30 years before Colton was born, then shared impossible-to-know details about each of them. He went on to explain numerous details about heaven and he continues to tell his story to whomever will listen to this day.

Knowing that there is a heaven and that you've been designed to end up there after you die has got to be one of the most profound and comforting realizations that a human can have. Talk about improving your health! I believe it with all my heart, and I live differently in light of my faith. I would, however, be straight-up lying if I said that I haven't ever had any doubts in the past and that now I have it all figured out. In fact, I have had serious doubts and have had to seek and search for the meaning of life and for some evidence of the existence of God.

In seeking the truth and trying to "prove" or "disprove" His existence, I've come to a stronger and deeper faith and belief in God. In my final analysis, what I realized was that we can't prove, explain, or understand everything in this life. It all boils down to trust. We must simply trust that God loves us, has a plan, and that it will all work out in the end. Trusting means that we let go of control, and in doing so, peace comes into our hearts. There's no real peace without total trust. Once found, that peace is a wellspring of health!

"PROVING" THE EXISTENCE OF GOD

I really like a particular scene, again, from the movie *Contact*, where the two main actors—a renegade "man of the cloth" played by Matthew McConaughey and a space scientist played by Jodie Foster—are discussing the existence of God. The scientist says, "Let me tell you about Occam's razor. It's a basic scientific principle that says, all things being equal, the simplest explanation tends to be the right one."

To which he replies, "Makes sense to me."

She goes on, "So which is more likely: that an all-powerful, mysterious God created the universe and then decided not to give any proof of His existence, or that He simply doesn't exist at all and we created Him so we wouldn't feel so small and alone?"

He replies, "I don't know…I can't imagine living in a world where God didn't exist. No—I wouldn't want to."

The scientist presses, "How do you know you're not deluding yourself? I mean, for me…I'd need proof."

Then, knowing that the scientist loved her father dearly before his death, he asks her, "Did you love your father?"

She immediately replies, "Yes…very much!"

He ends the conversation and leaves her in a state of silent pondering by simply challenging her, "Prove it." (I've got tears welling up in my eyes again.) He said it lovingly and it helped her see his point.

I thought, Whoa! That's such a good way of explaining it. I love science and I love understanding how things work and having a solid, undeniable, definitive answer for everything. However, there are just some things in this world that you can't see, or touch, or prove—but that doesn't change the fact that they're as *real* as they can be.

Listen, I totally get it. Way too many people have been deeply hurt by people in the church. In fact, most people have been offended or confused by something they've seen someone do in the "name" of religion. The thing is, God is *not* religion…that's a human creation. We can't confuse the failures and atrocities of religion with the heart of God. Humans are flawed and they do and say things that hurt others, but God loves.

Love is the most powerful force in the universe. You can't see it or touch it or measure it or prove it, but you can see the effect of love now and throughout history. As a boy, I was taught that God is love—that *God* and *love* are interchangeable words. So, like in the movie, where McConaughey's character highlighted that you can't prove that love exists, you can't prove that God exists either. Billy Graham, the spiritual advisor to many presidents of the United States has a very famous quote that sums it up nicely: "Can you see God? You haven't seen Him? I've never seen the wind. I see the effects of the wind, but I've never seen the wind. There's a mystery to it."[1] Even though we can't scientifically prove much about God or our faith, their effect on our lives, and, in turn, on our health, is profound.

There's so much more to explore than the existence of God, which can't be done by scientific methods. I encourage you to read more and continue to learn and grow. I do every day. As we seek out and learn more about God, our understanding grows, and this gives us increased faith.

TRUE LOVE AND FREE WILL

One of the most difficult things to wrap my head around has been that if there is a God, and if He is a loving God, then why does He allow bad things to happen, especially to good people? There, of course, is the obvious basic argument from the creation story that when man and woman disobeyed God in the garden ("the fall of man"), it disrupted the perfection that was intended to exist on the earth. That deviation from the Original Design created a series of linked events that led to everything from gene mutation to natural disasters.

However, there was a truth that crystallized in my mind, as I was going through a tough time in my own life, that has served to answer many questions and solidify my faith. I came to the realization that the greatest thing anyone could hope for on this earth was to give love and to receive love. Money, fame, power, sex, drugs, and yes, even rock 'n' roll can only satisfy for so long, and ultimately they all leave us feeling empty. They always have and they always will. True love, however, is what's at the center of the human experience. True love is what we all want, what we all need, and what we all are searching for. For it to truly be real love, it has to be freely given and can't be forced in any way.

If I paid actors large amounts of money to come and perform an elaborate skit, during which they tell me they love me, how loved would I truly feel? I'm going to go with—umm—not at all! It's fake, and I know it is! I paid them to pretend that they loved me. It's totally hollow and does nothing for me. However, when the people I interact with, especially family, stop what they're doing and of their own free will grab me by the face, look into my eyes, and say, "I love you!" and give me a big warm hug, I feel fantastic, and deeply and genuinely loved. That's true love. For love to be true and real and rich, it has to be unrehearsed by someone with free will to choose to give it or not to give it.

I thought that if God is out there, then He must also want to love and be loved back. If we're created in His image, then He surely understands and even shares much of what's in *our* hearts, as they were designed from His.

Luckily, nearly everyone on this planet can agree that we have a free will. I can choose to love or hate, eat healthy or junky food, be a positive person or a negative person, and, ultimately, I can choose to live or die. In order for true love to exist, there must be free will.

The issue with that, of course, is that the people He created, His own children, would have the ability to choose not only to love Him, but to hate Him, curse Him, or refuse to believe that He even exists. Wow. It must've been a heartbreaking realization for God. To have the ability to keep the ones you love from making dumb mistakes, but realizing that you must allow and even expect them to make horrible choices had to be the biggest challenge that He faced. God knew that free will would create problems as simple as broken hearts and "little" white lies, all the way down to disasters as awful as wars, mass murders, and plagues. It was a huge price to pay for true love to exist, but it was worth it.

God could've made us all robots. He could've made everything work out perfectly and no bad things would ever happen, especially not to "good" people. He could've programmed us to love Him and to act perfectly, but then it wouldn't be reality. It'd be a playback of some prerecorded, fake "reality" TV show that's *like* life, but has no soul, no thrill, no real happiness, and, of course, no true love. What would be the point in that? Robots can't ever fill the hole in the heart that only true love can fill. True love gives meaning to life.

People have always wanted to know the meaning of life. There are, in fact, many wonderful and amazing things that you can experience on this earth. You can climb the highest mountain, achieve great wealth or fame, win a race, overcome all of the obstacles, taste the most wonderful foods and drinks, see the most beautiful sites, hear the most beautiful music, and laugh until you cry. But all of those are empty in the end. At the heart of the matter is this: Without true love—the most amazing, pure, powerful force on earth—there would be no point to being here.

If I were stuck in a prison for life, and had no family or friends on the outside who loved me, and I had nothing but the four concrete walls to comfort me, I can't say that I could muster up the will to live for long. But if you put me in that same prison *with* my wife and kids, not only could I endure it but quite possibly, with their love to fuel me, I might be able to break down the walls and set us free. True love is powerful stuff!

If you're thinking to yourself that you don't have someone to love, or that no one loves you, then you're wrong. God always loves you and will always be there for you. On a human level, someone out there loves you too, or will love you in the future. You must simply trust that, in time, that person will find you, or you will find them, when the time is right. Some of you may need to allow yourself to be loved romantically, or even by a friend. You must first focus on being the person God created you to be, and everything else will come naturally.

ALL YOU NEED IS LOVE

I think the Beatles may have been right. Sing it with me! "♫All you need is love....♫" Love is the greatest gift you can give or receive. It's what we all search for, it's what we all need, and it's at the central core of faith. Without love, we cannot achieve the level of health we were designed to enjoy, because we were designed to love and be loved by God, as well as by others. Without love, we'd be in bad shape—our hearts would be empty and cold.

When people are in the hospital and their bodies are failing, with only a few moments to live, what do they want? A bicycle? A diamond ring? An award? A slice of pie? To be back at work? Nope. They want the love of close family and friends. Love is everything. When you think about it, some of the most absolutely beautiful and profound moments in life are when God is loving us, when we're loving God, when we're loving others, and when others are loving us. There's nothing sweeter in life than love.

I think about one of the most "loved" scriptures in the Bible. It's found in First Corinthians 13:1-8,13 AMP:

> If I speak with the tongues of men and of angels, but have not love, then I have become only a noisy gong or a clanging cymbal. And if I have *the gift of* prophecy and understand all mysteries, and all knowledge; and if I have all faith so that I can remove mountains, but do not have love…I am nothing. If I give all my possessions to feed *the poor*, and if I surrender my body to be burned, but do not have love, it does me no good at all.
>
> Love endures with patience *and* serenity, love is kind *and* thoughtful, and is not jealous *or* envious; love does not brag and is not proud *or* arrogant. It is not rude; it is not self-seeking, it is not provoked; it does not take into account a wrong *endured*. It does not rejoice at injustice, but rejoices with the truth.…Love bears all things, believes all things, hopes all things, endures all things.…
>
> Love never fails.
>
> And now there remain: faith, hope, love, these three; but the greatest of these is love.

What more can we say? Love is the greatest prize; it is the destination and the fuel to get there. Love is the reason behind all that we do. It is what designed us. Love is "it."

LOVE ISN'T JUST A FEELING

Why is love in a chapter about faith? Shouldn't it be under emotions? It certainly could be, but love isn't just a feeling; rather, it's the most important force in the universe. Love is what motivates people to do the most amazing things that have ever been accomplished, and it's our most prized possession as humans. We hear people say, "I don't care what happens—I could lose everything and I'd be okay as long as you love me."

God never stops loving us. God's love isn't something that comes and goes. It's not there just when we do something "good," and it doesn't go away when we've done something "bad." It doesn't matter what we've done; His love for us isn't based on what we've done, but on who we are. We're His children. When my kids act up, I might have feelings of disappointment or frustration, but it never touches my love for them. There's nothing that any of us can do to earn or deserve God's love. It was there from the beginning, before our first breath, and nothing will ever change His love for us.

When my daughters were born, I didn't wait a few years for them to achieve some things to see if I was going to love them. I wasn't waiting to analyze their behavior or accomplishments before love developed in my heart for them. That love was there even before they were born. From the moment my wife and I knew she was pregnant, my heart was forever caught up in an intense feeling of love for them. Nothing will ever change that. Knowing that God loves us even more than what I felt for my kids is a total game changer! Sadly, not everyone believes that God loves us.

I've talked with so many patients who have a skewed idea of who God is. Many people see God as an angry taskmaster who is waiting to strike them down when they do wrong. Others think that God is a distant ghostly being in the clouds who's unapproachable and barely even knows or cares that they exist. For me, as I understand more and more about how the body works, I see a Designer who passionately cares about every intimate detail of my body, mind, and soul. If He designed me, then why wouldn't He love and care for me at least like an earthly father loves his children? Artists who design masterpieces don't step on them or toss them to the side. No, they treat them with great care and give them a place of honor in their homes. They show them off to all who come by because they're proud of what they've made. They love them.

I love being a dad for a lot of reasons, but one really cool thing is how my relationship with my kids reminds me of God's relationship with me. I can't truly express how much I love my kids and how, without hesitation, I would lay down my life for them if necessary. How much more must God love us if we can feel such intense love here on earth in a human relationship?

Most of human love is conditional. It depends on how we're treated. God's love is independent of how we treat Him. His love is much deeper. It's the fuel that our souls use to flourish and be healthy. When we find God's love, we have a peace in our hearts that gives us hope, happiness, and purpose. Without it, there's only an emptiness and sadness that will absolutely wreck our health. God's love heals all wounds and is available to us, whether or not we choose to believe it and accept it.

KEEP LOVE AS THE FOCUS

When I was little, we used to sing a song in church that said, "They will know we are Christians by our love." Sadly, we all fail in showing love as often and as completely as we should or could. Often, people will say that Christians are hypocrites because of how they act. I see how they could feel that way, considering how some people act...even me at times. I'd say that it's more a matter of failing to do what they know to be right, rather than thinking they're better than anyone else.

That would be like calling me a hypocrite for eating a chocolate chip cookie because I'm a nutritionist. It's much simpler than that. I just caved in a moment of weakness (or maybe it was my splurge meal!). I know better, but I failed. I don't pretend to be better than anyone else, I simply understand which foods help my body be the healthiest it can be.

Truthfully, we all should be more concerned with working on our own personal issues instead of pointing our finger at others. One scripture says to worry about the plank in your own eye before telling someone else about the speck in theirs (see Matthew 7:1-5). Isn't that so true? I have enough issues of my own—I don't have the time or the right to point out other people's problems. I need only to show them love, grace, and acceptance. Now, if they ask, then that's a different story—I'd be happy to tell 'em! (I'm kidding.)

I love the story in the Bible where the woman who'd been caught in adultery was being dragged out to be stoned by the religious people. But Jesus said, "He who is without sin among you, let him throw a stone at her first" (John 8:7). Needless to say, they all dropped their stones and walked away. It's not up to us to judge or point out someone else's failures. Our only job is to love. Everything else is between that person and God. And guess what? The Bible says that He's quick to forgive—all we have to do is ask Him. Healing of your soul is only a short talk with God away. There's no good reason to put it off any longer.

WHO'S RIGHT AND WHO'S WRONG?

There are certainly details about practicing faith that would be argued by even churches of the same faith and denominations on opposite street corners of the same town. What's worse is that people in the same church and members of the same family will routinely disagree about their faith, for crying out loud. Let's not go down *that* road. Family feuds are messy business.

Are any of us audacious enough to believe that we're the only ones who've truly figured out God? Think about it. Just within the Christian faith, if each church has its own set of beliefs and interpretations about the Word of God, and believes that everyone else is wrong, then they have about a one in 3.7 million chance that they are right. (There are proposed to be 3.7 million different congregations in the world.) When we get to heaven, do we really believe that all the Baptists will be in one corner, all the Catholics in another, and all the Jews in another? I think not. Why would God reveal Himself and His true path to only one specific church?

It seems more logical that if we believe in God, then we have to believe that He left His Word open to *some* degree of interpretation, or He would've spelled it out a lot more specifically and given us fewer parables and generalities. While there are certainly some things that are so clear that they don't leave themselves open to much interpretation, there are plenty of things that aren't. Again, let's not focus on our differences of faith. Remember that exactly what you believe is likely different from what everyone else in your church believes, and your church is just one of 3.7 million in the world today. Let's focus on what is believed by nearly all of us.

As I said earlier in the book, the fact is that roughly 90% of the world's population believes in God, a Creator who designed all people and all things. He still exists today and loves us dearly, regardless of who we are or what we've done. To those of you who are reading this book and who don't believe in one almighty God, Creator of the universe, then I hope you're at least able to glean some helpful information from what you're reading and are able to keep an open mind to the overall principles of what I'm trying to get across.

Regardless of your faith, my true heart's desire is to help people lead the healthiest, happiest life they possibly can. I've listened to some of the greatest doctors, scientists, motivational speakers, coaches, pastors, and philosophers of our day. I didn't always share or agree with all of their beliefs or theories either, but I was always able to decipher wisdom when I heard it. I was able to take little bits and pieces of information that helped shape what I believe, to boost my knowledge, and make me who I am today.

Let me make this statement bold and clear: Never tune others out simply because they don't understand or express *their* faith the exact same way as you! So please stick with me if you feel like we don't see eye to eye, because most of us have trouble agreeing with anyone about all aspects of faith anyway. There's still a lot of good information in this book that can truly help you attain a greater level of health in this world. I've seen it greatly benefit thousands of people—it might just help you too!

THE POWER OF PRAYER

Every religion on the planet communicates with God in some way or another. The most common way, of course, is through prayer, but some religions believe that communication with God can only be done through a designated high-ranking leader of the religion. The exciting thing about Christianity, however, and what I believe to be consistent with the true heart of God, is that anyone can talk to Him directly at any time. That is extremely comforting.

When my daughters close their eyes, fold their hands, and begin speaking to God, He hears them and is delighted with their prayers. The cool thing is that we don't have to close our eyes or fold our hands to pray. My kids are simply copying what they've seen. Actually, I talk to God all the time. I talk to God while writing, adjusting patients, working out, hiking, driving, and pretty much anytime I'm not engaged directly in a conversation with another person.

In a book called *90 Minutes in Heaven*, a pastor tells his story of being pronounced dead at the scene of a horrific auto accident. A passing car stopped, and the man inside, who was also a pastor, felt led to pray for the "dead man." He was told by several paramedics that it was too late and that there was no point. The man persisted until they allowed him to go to the crushed car with the victim inside and pray. An hour and a half after his heart stopped in the crash, the man came back from heaven to continue living his life on this earth. His story and details of heaven are amazing, but I'm pretty sure he and his family were glad for prayer.

Surprisingly, many studies have been done on the ability of prayer to affect the outcome of health in the human body. This is clearly a subject that we're all interested in, but it's discarded by science as invalid. The results are truly remarkable and speak for themselves.

One of the most well-known and quoted studies on the power of prayer was done at San Francisco General Hospital's Coronary Care Unit. Between August of 1982 and May of 1983, 393 patients in the Coronary Care Unit participated in a double-blind trial assessing the effects of prayer.[2] By random computer selection, half of the patients were chosen to receive prayer while the other half would not. None of the patients had any way of knowing to which group they had been assigned.

In the final analysis of the study, patients who had received prayer were healthier overall versus those who had not. Compared to the control group, the patients who were prayed for had less need for antibiotics, CPR, diuretics, and mechanical ventilators. Amazingly, the patients who were prayed for also had fewer occurrences of a serious condition called pulmonary edema (which can lead to heart failure), and there were fewer deaths in that group too. The doctors and nurses were all astonished. That is the power of prayer.

Another way that prayer affects your health is simply by how it affects the physiology or function of your brain. When you pray, the hypothalamus is stimulated, which is the part of the brain that controls chemicals released to decrease blood pressure, muscle tension, and heart rate, as well as to increase the capacity of the lungs to carry oxygen.

One study conducted by Duke University Medical Center followed over 4,000 participants over the age of 65. The study found that those who pray and attend religious services on a weekly basis had lower blood pressure than their counterparts who didn't pray or attend religious services. Interestingly, they found that the more the person prayed and the more regularly they attended church, the lower their blood pressure.

In fact, the study found that these people were 40% less likely to have high blood pressure than those who did not attend religious services, pray, or study the Bible.[3] The president of the National Institute for Health Care Research in Rockville, Maryland, coauthored the study and said, "Faith brings a calming state which helps decrease nervousness and anxiety with coping with day-to-day stress."[4]

Often, prayer is seen as a panic button when you need something from God really badly. That, of course, is a perfect time to connect with Him, just as we want to hear from our children when they are hurting or in need. However, don't we love to talk to our kids when they're happy or excited too? Of course! In fact, those might be some of our favorite conversations with our kids. In a similar way, God wants to have these kinds of conversations with us too. They create a rich relationship and help strengthen our faith and health.

Here's "proof" that prayer can benefit your health in the good times: A really cool study conducted by the Virginia Commonwealth University Medical College in Richmond analyzed the lives of 1,902 sets of twins. It turned out that those individuals committed to spiritual lives tended to have lower rates of addiction, depression, and divorce than their twins. The study linked their active, regular involvement in a spiritual community to their overall stability and health.[5]

In general, it's been found that prayer can change things when nothing else could be done. You'll often hear people say, "All we can do is pray." It almost sounds like it's not much, but prayer is powerful and shouldn't be a last-ditch effort when all is lost. Prayer should be one of the *first* things we do to connect with God on a daily basis.

WE CAN'T EARN IT

None of us are going to impress God with who we are or what we've done. We can't earn our way to heaven. Can we ever do "enough" good things to get in? How could we possibly gauge that? What's the measuring stick?

For example, can we pray long enough, hard enough, eloquently enough, with big enough words or enough memorized Scripture to impress Him and personally achieve His love and the gifts of complete forgiveness and eternal life? Nope. Not a chance. It's not a secret formula.

None of us deserve God's love; we only get it because of grace. God saves us, loves us, and calls us by name because we're His children whom He specifically designed. It's not because of what we do or what we say. When you think about it, it really takes a lot of pressure off of us when we realize this.

Of course, we should always do our best to do the "right things." But we also need to remember that His love is there for us independent of our performance, whether a great achievement or a horrible failure. What a relief! Honestly, if we thought we had to actually earn our way to heaven, it would be exhausting. Fear, insecurity, and uncertainty would rule our lives. God doesn't want to judge us for our past; He wants to free us up for our future.

Something amazing happens when we combine our faith with God's willingness to heal.

ASK, SEEK, AND KNOCK

My mom always told me when I was growing up that if I wanted something, all I needed to do was ask. What's the worst that can happen? "The answer could be no!" I'd say. "Ah, but it could be yes! You'll never know unless you ask," she'd reply. The Bible says that if we ask, we'll receive; if we seek we'll find; and when we knock, the door will be opened. Sometimes we simply need to muster up the faith to give it a try, whatever the need, whether big or small.

One of my favorite stories of faith as it relates directly to health is in Mark 5:25-32. There are so many cool points to the story. It's the story of the woman who'd been plagued with a blood disease for 12 years. She'd been suffering for a long time, under the care of doctors, spending all she had, only to grow continually worse.

She fought through the crowd to touch just the hem of Jesus's garment. When she finally touched it, she was instantly healed. Jesus stopped and said, "Who touched Me?" Now this is quite peculiar. He was walking through and surrounded by a crowd of people—hundreds if not thousands of people were pressing in around Him. In fact, His disciples draw this to His attention, but Jesus said, "No, someone *touched* Me and I felt power come out of My body." Well, that's a different story. Notice that He was not specifically focused on healing her at that moment—she simply reached out and touched Him.

He had already said and shown that He was willing to heal people, but *she* had faith that all she needed to do was touch a small piece of His robe. That wasn't His stipulation, but what she believed in her heart would heal her. God reveals to each of us what *we* should do, specifically and individually.

The woman came forward, and He proclaimed, "Daughter, your faith has healed you. Go in peace and be freed from your suffering" (Mark 5:34 NIV). Faith is an incredibly powerful thing. Something amazing happens when we combine our faith with God's willingness to heal. We only need to believe and act on our faith.

Most of us have had to face some serious health issues in our lives or in the life of a close loved one. It's in these times where we need to know what we believe and be ready to put our faith into action. People may say that they have no faith or don't believe in God, but it's interesting what they do and say when they've been given extremely dire news, possibly even that they have only a short time to live. It changes everything and forces them to reevaluate what they believe mighty quickly. That moment when we're faced with our mortality and an uncertainty of life after death is when all of us call out to God. That's no accident. It's part of our Original Design. We are prewired to call home, to call upon our heavenly Father. It's our only lifeline and the only one we need.

Listen. I've got great news for you. God is the same yesterday, today, and forever. He has designed you and everything in this universe. He loves you and cares about you more than you'll ever know. Nothing you do can ever change that.

Seek Him and a deeper knowledge of all that He has designed for you. Ask Him whatever it is that you know in your heart that you need to know. Knock on His door, and He will open it. Your heart, your health, and your life will never be the same. There's an unbelievable peace waiting for you. There are no requirements, no fees, and no obligations. It's just you and Him right now. Whether or not you have faith in God, He's always there for you and *He* has faith in *you*.

CONCLUSION

CHAPTER 15

INPUT/OUTPUT

All of life is about flow. In order for there to be output, there must be input. It's an essential concept of the Original Design. Things must go *through* you. If there's no flow, then there's stagnation, dysfunction, illness, and eventual death. Would you rather drink from a stagnant puddle or a flowing mountain stream? All of life is dependent on flow—absorption of nutrients in digestion, nervous system function, joint hydration and movement, oxygen assimilation, creating and maintaining relationships, development of inborn talent or ideas, fulfilling your purpose, good health, the operation of every cell in your body—life itself is critically dependent on flow. Flow depends on input and output.

What we put in our minds, bodies, hearts, and spirits is so incredibly important because it determines what comes out or what the "outcome" will be in our health. So, in some ways, our bodies are machines like any other machine: we are input/output machines. You often hear that computers are input/output machines, meaning that whatever you put into the computer is then available to come out. The only thing, in fact, that can come out of it is what was put into it. In other words, if you don't first put something in, then you can't get it out. Deep, right?

However, before we go any further, I want to make a significant distinction here. I've heard it said that "what goes in *must* come out," playing on the old phrase, "What goes up must come down." I think this is absolutely untrue and is, in fact, a defeatist attitude. This would suggest that if you were abused, you have no choice but to be an abuser yourself. That is complete bull! Let's say that you saw unhealthy eating habits growing up and that information is stored in your database; you don't have to repeat those bad habits. You *can* make different and wiser choices in your own life.

Don't let anyone tell you differently. You have free will and *you* determine your own destiny, not your past! What has happened to you in the past may be something that you can't forget and something that you learn from, but it certainly doesn't determine what you'll do, what you'll say, or who you'll be in the future. Now that we have that clear, let's move on with the idea.

WHAT COMES OUT MUST FIRST GO IN

In other words, you can't get data out of a computer that you haven't already "preloaded" into it. You can't recall a memory if it never happened. You won't be able to lift something heavy if you haven't already prepared your muscles to have the physical strength they need to do the job. You can't give someone your time if you don't have time to give. You won't handle a situation that you come to in life as well as you could unless you have already trained to know what to do when that situation arises. I know this might sound obvious, but stick with me for a minute.

The Original Design is for all of us to be able to handle what this life brings—mentally, physically, chemically, and spiritually. You were specifically designed for a specific purpose with free will and the ability to choose. The key is that what you put *in* allows you to get *out* the results that you were designed to experience.

Back to the old phrase we heard when we were kids: "You are what you eat." Well, most of us would agree that this is true to a great extent. If we eat junk food, our bodies are going to become junky, and we'll begin to gain weight, have sickness, and experience dysfunction and pain. This is no accident. However, if we put the right food into our bodies, there's a much greater chance that we're going to have health, normal function, very little pain, and a much more enjoyable life.

You can't respond appropriately with how you act or speak, unless you've already input the right tools into the "database" of your brain and heart.

In the same way, if we fill our minds full of negative information like violence, hate, discord, sadness, anger, or any other negative emotion that we can experience as humans, then we're going to be full of *those* emotions or data. When we're pressed in our lives, we'll often respond with all of those same emotions, but we don't have to.

This "data" or information comes from anything that we *allow* into our minds and hearts. This would be by the music that we listen to, what we watch on TV, the newspapers we read, what we look at on the Internet, what we hear on the radio, the people we surround ourselves with, and what they say. Basically, who you are is typically a by-product of everything that you surround yourself with, or what you've been subjected to. But again, remember that it doesn't have to be that way. Once you're an adult, and "out of the house," *you* choose what goes in, and this affects what comes out.

The big idea here is this: You can't respond appropriately with how you act or speak, unless you've already input the right tools into the "database" of your brain and heart. The great news is that you can reprogram or overwrite the bad stuff that was put there first. You just have to start inputting the right "data" that's good and uplifting and wise and noble and positive and healthy.

People often wonder why they make the wrong choices. I would argue that it's not just that they were "raised" wrong or bad things happened to them. You might have had poor parenting in childhood, but if you reprogram your brain and your heart with new information, that leads you to think and act and speak differently, then you've found the secret to making better choices.

This is where you become powerful and take control over your life and choose to do what is right, because now you know what is right. As they say, knowledge is power! Then, of course, you must act on this newfound knowledge. Remember: Wisdom is knowledge applied (acted upon).

When patients ask me a question about their health, often the answer is way longer than what we have time for. The whole point of writing this book was so that I could help equip people with information that can completely change the course of their lives…for the better. Learning and then applying the knowledge you've gained in the last 14 chapters (and what's available in thousands of other books full of great information) is what can fill your database with the "tools" to be the healthiest you can be. Your database is being reprogrammed with the right info even now!

CHOOSE THE RIGHT INPUT

I am so pumped up about this principle; it's just so solid and absolutely foundational to me! Everything that I think of or have applied this principle to seems to fall right in line with the Original Design. God designed every single cell in our bodies and He provided everything that we need to live the most vital lives that this world can offer. However, when we choose to fill our lives full of junk, whether it's informational, emotional, or dietary, we stray from that design and we won't be happy or healthy. If I only ever fill a cookie jar with cow patties, it doesn't matter how many times I open and close the jar, I'll always pull out a turd—not a cookie. Are ya with me?

Every time you see others who are going through a challenging time in their health, you can almost always trace it back and find the point at which they began to veer from the true path they were designed to have been on.

Somewhere or another, they have made a poor choice in one or more areas of health. When it comes to achieving optimal health, we have to look at all the areas of our lives that affect our health. This is what the gist of this entire book has been about. You have to analyze what has been put in to explain what's coming out.

We have to look at what we're eating, the information, people, and things that we're allowing to influence us, the amount of rest and exercise we're getting, the amount of time spent laughing and playing, and whether we're devoting ourselves on a regular basis to time with God, and family and friends. So often the *quality* of our lives is directly related to how closely we adhere to the Original Design. Replacing what God has for us with a cheap counterfeit will always result in disappointment and less than the best outcome. Peace and comfort come when we realize that we don't have to reinvent what was already designed for us. It's so simple.

If you've read the previous chapters of this book, you know that I'm not saying that there should be no progress, or that there should be no technology, or that we shouldn't try to create anything. We should constantly create new art, new music, new inventions, new ways to love people, new recipes, new ideas, and new ways to improve the lives of people. That, in fact, is part of the Original Design—to create and invent and change.

The important thing to understand here is that we simply don't want to alter our food, water, soil, bodies, relationships, minds, sleep, or any parts of the Original Design of our core needs. Again, I'm glad we invented forks, indoor plumbing, guitars, warm clothes, organic dark chocolate-covered almonds, and soft pillows. You get the idea.

**People are sick and tired
of being sick and tired.**

SICK AND TIRED

When I talk to individual patients in my office, or when I speak to large groups, I hear the same thing over and over again: People are sick and tired of being sick and tired. They're unhappy, unhealthy, and not enjoying life. They may try to trace it back to any number of issues, like not being born into a family that has money, not having a spouse who treats them well, not having the genetically perfect body, not having parents who love them, or not being born on the right side of the tracks. They have a million reasons why they don't have vibrant health and peace in their hearts. All those are important and have to be taken into account, but you can't change them. There's so much more value in focusing on what you can change.

I've heard it from poor migrant workers to CEOs of Fortune 500 companies, and everywhere in between—your financial or social position just doesn't matter…*anyone* can be unhealthy and unhappy.

Just recently I had a perfect illustration of this one morning in my practice. A frustrated guy came in to see me who drove a $100,000 supercar, lived in a massive home, had been financially successful in several jobs, and had a beautiful wife and kids. Every sentence that he uttered was negative and whiney. By the time we were through with his appointment, I felt mentally and physically exhausted.

Right after him, a happy single guy came in who was homeless and driving a junker car that he'd been given. As this world sees it, he didn't have much to his name. However, we had the greatest emotional and spiritual conversation during his appointment, which ended in a hug and left me feeling happy and optimistic about the world. Which one was healthier?

The self-talk and information that these two guys put into their minds and hearts were totally different. One always listened to, read, and watched negative things and made negative statements that produced a sad existence, while the other guy rarely let negative input into his brain and heart, and made positive statements despite his situation.

Our level of peace and happiness and how we affect others is more dependent on the attitude we choose to have than it is on the circumstances we're experiencing. You don't have to act sick and tired, even if life is treating you unfairly. I'm here to tell you that you can quickly make positive changes in your life starting right now, today. This will begin a transformation process that will bring you closer and closer, day by day, to what was originally designed for you to be, do, and have. It's your birthright to have a life of health, happiness, peace in your heart, and a satisfaction that you may have never believed was available to you in this world.

Am I promising a perfect existence, without any pain, suffering, frustration, or challenges while lounging in a mansion and being chauffeured everywhere you go? No, of course not. There's no such thing, and anyone who offers that is deceiving you. In fact, we're guaranteed that there will be hardships, trials, heartbreak, frustration, and even persecution in this world.

What is possible, however, is something far better than what you're dealing with or feeling like right now. Every step that you take to get in alignment with the Original Design for your life that God made from the beginning, the closer you will be to living the life for which you are longing, the life that you were meant to live.

WORDS HAVE POWER

As I was writing this particular section of the book, I was dictating it to my computer through voice recognition software on a trip to Houston with my friend Rick. As we were traveling, he and I were discussing the negative things we so often hear people say around us on a regular basis, even members of our own families and close friends: "I just can't lose weight," or "Dang it. I just can't ever seem to get ahead," or "I'm always getting sick," or "I'm so tired." They might even say something like, "My husband is such an idiot!" or "I'm a big fat slob."

What they're saying to themselves is an affirmation that they repeat over and over again about each of those various issues. Rick added in that "they're reinforcing and making an agreement in their hearts with the very thing that they're disgusted with." And he's so right. This has to stop, and it has to stop now.

I once heard a pastor say that you can follow any sentence that you say about yourself or about something in your life with this ending, "and that's the way I want it." The person is saying then, "I just can't seem to lose weight, *and that's the way I want it.*" Can you see how that changes the feeling of that statement? Voicing a negative thought tells your heart and mind what to expect and focus on and, soon enough, it becomes a reality.

Hold on. Let's go a little further here because this is so important. Let me ask you a question: What's the point in stating something in your mind, or especially out loud, that is absolutely contrary to what you *want* to see happen in your life? There's absolutely no point. What do you gain? Absolutely nothing. There's not one good thing that comes from speaking negatively about yourself or your situation—so stop it!

**If you say that you want something
to change, start by changing what you say!**

When have you ever heard of anyone beating cancer by saying, "Ya know, I guess I'm just gonna die. This thing is gonna be the end of me. Oh well, it's all over"? Do people who think and speak to themselves like this actually go on to beat cancer? Rarely. Rather, the story you always hear is the person who gets diagnosed with cancer and then says, "I am not going to die! I'm going to beat this thing, no matter what I do!"

I have a friend named Matt who was diagnosed with testicular cancer as a young man. It's the most common cancer in males ages 15 to 34. He had surgery and had one of his testicles removed. His whole world came to a screeching halt. He could've gotten depressed and given up, but he fought it with everything in him and told himself he wouldn't let it slow him down. Since then, he got married to a beautiful woman, had two kids, started the Testicular Cancer Foundation, and is helping thousands of young men all across the world in their battles with cancer!

Proverbs 18:21 (NIV) says, "The tongue has the power of life and death." That's a pretty serious statement. We can't just throw around lightly the words that come out of our mouths. If you say that you want something to change, start by changing what you say! As I began to learn about how powerful our words are, whether they are positive or negative, I couldn't believe the effect they have. What you say about yourself or your situation can never be underestimated.

It's important to speak what you want to see. Joel 3:10 tells us, "Let the weak say, 'I am strong.'" There's something powerful about what we say, even more powerful than what we think. Sometimes, simply encouraging another person with what we say can be the difference in his or her personal road to health. Proverbs 16:24 (NIV) says, "Gracious words are a honeycomb, sweet to the soul and healing to the bones."

Think about the words that come out of your mouth before you say them, and judge them as to whether or not they are declaring what you want to see happen in your life, and if they benefit you or those around you. Many times our words are simply describing what we're currently seeing happen or even describing something that we fear will come to pass. There's no point in stating the obvious! That doesn't change anything, and it certainly doesn't help your attitude or outlook on the situation.

My wife and I have a little joke with each other that when one of us says something that's blatantly obvious, the other person will make a little trumpet sound, "Der der DER!" This is supposed to represent the announcing of the arrival of our fictitious superhero, Captain Obvious, who's always stating the obvious. We will both laugh, and it serves as a gentle reminder to let our words have value and not simply state something that's clear to everyone.

Take, for instance, if one of us is sweating and struggling as we work on a project that's difficult to do and the other one exclaims, "That looks really hard!" The other person makes the little trumpet noise and we will both laugh, thinking to ourselves, "Thank you, Captain Obvious, for not helping…at all!" What we should say, what you hear coaches say to their teams, and what good bosses say to their staff members on a regular basis, are words of encouragement and positivity. Have you ever heard coaches say to their players at halftime, "Man, we're really awful! We are way behind. Y'all are playing horribly, and there's no chance we're gonna win this game." Of course not! Are you kidding me? That would be the worst coach in the entire world.

You're much more likely to hear them say something like, "I know what it looks like on the outside, but I know this one thing, team. I know what you're capable of. I know your heart. We've come back from bigger deficits than this. You have it within you to dig deep and overcome all the challenges that we've been having. The only thing that stands between you and victory is believing in yourself and knowing that you were created for this moment, right here, right now. You have the ability. You have the talent. You know what to do. Now let's go out there and do this! Let's win!"

Hey, that was pretty good! I shoulda been a coach! That's the kind of stuff that we should be saying to ourselves every single day. As a Christian, I was taught that we can overcome any obstacle through Jesus Christ. We were designed to overcome, but we can't overcome when all we do is talk about and focus on how we're failing. When we use words to encourage and build up ourselves and others, we all begin to win.

I'm convinced that if you plant seeds of positivity and hope and joy in people's lives, you'll reap an incredible harvest of those same things in your own life. The whole "Pass it on!" phenomenon is real. Kindness, happiness, and joy are contagious. Plant those good seeds every chance you get.

THE BEST YOU IS JUST AROUND THE CORNER

Your greatest level of health may be just around the corner! Very soon you could have the most physical health, emotional stability, spiritual strength, peace, and joy in your life that you've ever had, simply by changing what you put inside of your body, mind, and heart. Starting today, begin your journey with just one little step, and when you do you'll be able to take two steps tomorrow, then three steps the next day, and so on. It won't be an overnight transformation, but it'll be faster than you think.

======

Wisdom is knowledge applied.

======

This journey will always include increasing what you know. You've heard it said here and other places numerous times that knowledge is power. I believe that to be true. The Bible says that "above all things" we are to get knowledge and wisdom (see Proverbs 4:7). As I said earlier, wisdom is knowledge applied. But before you can apply that knowledge, you have to learn it. This goes back to the idea that I started this chapter with, which is, "You have to put in you what you hope to later get out."

For many of you, you've already begun your journey by reading this book, and you've likely read other books that are also helping to build your knowledge database. Hopefully, you're turning that knowledge into wisdom by beginning to apply some of the principles that you've learned. For all of us, the journey continues.

We need to fill our lives with, first and foremost, a strong relationship with God. We have to trust Him and His Word, ask Him for guidance on who He designed us to be, and then to show us the steps to take to achieve that goal. This has rapid results that will quickly lay a firm foundation upon which to build our health. We also need to read, watch, and study more resources that guide us on our paths, and we need to spend more time with people we want to be like.

Make no mistake about it: *You* are no mistake! You're an original. You were created for a specific purpose. There's no one else on this planet who is like you or who is capable of doing what you were designed to do. Just because you may have wandered from the path that you were designed to be on doesn't mean that you can't get right back on track.

In fact, I've seen so many people turn their lives around and begin to experience the kind of health that they had always wanted but maybe thought was never possible. If you'll embrace the ideas in this book, seek out more knowledge and the wisdom in God's Word, I believe that you'll *quickly* be on your way toward becoming who you were made to be according to the Original Design.

ACCENTUATE THE POSITIVE

As I talk with patients, it's so funny to me how many of them will ask, "How do you stay so happy? You seem to be happy all of the time." For one thing, happiness is a choice. There's so much darkness in this world, so choose to be a light. Another thing is that it's really easy to be happy when you simply ignore all of the negative circumstances that are surrounding you. It sounds incredibly simple, but it's true and it's a key to being happy.

There's no value in focusing on the things in your life that aren't going well, or aren't going the way that you intended them to go. I always try to focus on and "live in" the positive areas in my life. God may have a good reason for what you're going through that you can't see...yet.

We've all heard some version of the story about how Thomas Edison, when asked why he hadn't been able to get any results when trying to invent a new battery, said, "I have gotten a lot of results! I know several thousand things that won't work."[1] He learned from what didn't work and focused on what did. That's a skill that's universal among people who succeed in any area of life, whether it's in their businesses or their marriages, or athletes in their particular sport—it's all the same.

Most of them will tell you that when something didn't go the way they intended it, or that they experienced some kind of failure, they simply took anything they could learn from that experience and moved on to whatever was next. Wallowing in failure or disappointment changes nothing. The one thing that you can be assured of is that if you stop seeking "it," you'll never find it. But learning from mistakes and taking the next step, with a *positive* attitude of gratitude, always moves you toward your goal.

Life is absolutely too short to waste time on people, places, or things that bring you down, separating you from your Original Design. If you repeatedly find yourself caught up in a negative feeling, train of thought, relationship, or situation, then isolate whatever it is and eliminate it as quickly as possible. Listen, I totally understand that some things may not be easily dismissed and may require some time to eliminate. That's okay. At least you've determined what the problem is in that area and you can now create a positive plan to fix it.

WHAT YOU THINK DETERMINES YOUR BELIEFS

When you think about it, all of us make decisions based off the knowledge that we have in our brains, which comes from our experiences, things we were taught by our parents, what we learned in school, read, heard, or otherwise accumulated in some way over time. The sum of all of that knowledge determines what we believe.

The greatest travesty that can ever befall you is for you to make an agreement that you can't do it, whatever "it" is. Whether you believe you can or believe you can't, you're probably right. However, you can't believe in something of which you don't have knowledge. As it pertains to *health*, we have to first build our knowledge by learning the right foods to eat, the right kind and amount of exercise to do, and the right thought patterns to have. Then the belief that we're capable of achieving health will follow.

Sadly, though, some of the knowledge that we learned was just plain bad. It was false knowledge that became false belief. We then acted out of that false belief, and it took us away from our Original Design. The wrong beliefs are from "stinkin' thinkin'," and that junk must be removed before we can move forward. Many people have been taught the wrong things for nearly their entire lives and therefore believe the wrong things about themselves, diet, faith, or nearly anything in the world.

Many of us have been so influenced by what we've learned from commercials, read in newspapers and magazines, or seen on TV shows and the Internet that we've become very self-assured in our wrong beliefs. Unfortunately, many of those beliefs are based on knowledge that was simply propaganda fed to us in order to get us to buy a product or think a certain way so that we would act in a way that was beneficial to someone else's agenda. Potato chip and prescription ads are *not* full of information to build up our health—they exist only to sell chips and drugs.

We have to deliberately input information into our brains' databases that helps us grow and believe in positive ways and steers our output toward our Original Design.

CHAPTER 16

THE BIG PICTURE

PERSPECTIVE

There are so many times I wish I could have some kind of giant reset button that would instantly give me the appropriate perspective and remind me of just how blessed I truly am. This magical button would remind me how privileged I am to live in the country that I do and to have all the freedoms that I have. With this button, I'd be able to see the big picture and be completely aware of the value of my family, my friends, my ability to worship freely, to practice my profession, to own my home, and the opportunity I have to create my own destiny.

Most of us don't wonder where our next meal will come from, if our clothes will hold together one more day, if we will have a roof over our head tonight, or if we'll even have the peace and quiet to get a good night's rest and be safe while we're sleeping. Most of us are even fortunate enough to have family and friends surrounding us who can lift us up when we're down. If we were able to have instant recall and hold all of that information and have it be fresh and at the forefront of our minds when we make decisions to act or speak, we might do things a little bit differently.

I'm reminded of the story of the lady who got on an airplane with her son one day. The little boy was acting a little bit rowdy, and so as she walked down the aisle, people avoided eye contact with her, as we all do, praying that she and her son would not sit next to them. As she got closer to the back of the plane, it became clear that there was only one row with two seats left. It happened to be right next to a weary businessman who'd been having a tough day and just wanted some peace and quiet.

As the lady and her kid took their seats, the boy's rowdiness intensified. Over the course of the next hour, it grew to a feverish pitch, hitting a peak when the boy knocked over the businessman's coffee, spilling it onto his lap and all over his paperwork. The woman had seemed to be oblivious to all of her son's activities, including the spill, which was simply too much for the man to remain silent.

In a moment of disbelief and rage, he turned to the woman and said, "Ma'am, can you please control your kid?" She snapped out of a blank stare and apologized to him, "I'm so sorry, sir," she said. "As I was getting on the airplane, I found out that my husband was killed in a car accident, and I've been trying to figure out how to tell my son that his daddy is dead."

Of course, immediately the businessman has complete forgiveness for her, puts his paperwork away, and even offers to read the boy a book and entertain him for the rest of the flight so that she can have some time to think. His initial judgement of the woman was that she was a horrible mother and a completely unaware person. However, as he got all of the information about her situation, his perspective changed dramatically and it immediately changed his attitude.

The man went from anger and frustration to sympathy and understanding, taking it as far as even trying to help her out. Wow! What a difference it makes when we have all the facts. We've all done it. It's human nature I suppose, but it's a good lesson when trying not to judge someone.

PRAYING FOR FORKS

One good practice to do daily in order to get a better perspective is to start off your day with prayer. It might benefit you to write down some points as a reminder of what to pray about. Praying for perspective is a really good way to hit that reset button each day. I often pray that God would allow me to have a big-picture mindset and not get too caught up in the minor details.

I'll also often pray that God allows me to see the "forks in the road." At many points throughout a day, we have an opportunity to choose one of several actions, responses, or attitudes concerning nearly anything in life. And whichever fork in the road we choose to take will have different outcomes.

My wife and I tell this to our kids all the time, and just recently our youngest daughter, Katie, decided she didn't want to watch Longhorn football with the family and sulked toward her bedroom alone. We sweetly told her that it was her choice, but that we'd love to have her with us and we'd miss her. She went to her room anyway and shut the door in a huff. About five minutes later she walked into the room where we were watching TV and we all rejoiced. I asked her why she changed her mind and she said something that made me so proud and made my wife cry. (Okay, I had a small tear too.)

She said, "I thought about it and I was at a fork in the road, Daddy. If I stayed in my room, I'd be sad, alone, and have no fun. If I came in here, I'd be with my family, I'd have fun, and I might get a special treat!" It's such a sweet story that perfectly illustrates the ability that we have as humans to pause and weigh out the options or consequences of our actions for anything we do in our lives.

For instance, when someone speeds by and cuts you off in traffic, you can respond in one of many ways: You can give him or her a common hand gesture that points the way to heaven and yell something colorful, or you can consider that there might be an emergency, pray for that person, and just let it go. The powerful option is to pray for the perspective that allows you to recognize the "fork in the road" at the instant it happens, or even before it happens. Then you can pause for a moment to choose a wise response.

Praying for the right perspective goes hand in hand with choosing the correct attitude which will develop peace in your life. The alternative is that you have a knee-jerk reaction that's not very well thought through and could have some pretty negative repercussions as a result.

Once, when I lived in Dallas for chiropractic school, I left a gross anatomy lab and began to drive home. As I was heading down the freeway, I had to take evasive action and swerve out of my lane to avoid being hit by another car that wasn't paying attention. As I did this, I made a tight squeeze in front of a car that was lowered, had music blaring, and was full of teenage boys who didn't see what happened. They weren't very fond of my actions and got right on my tail. This annoyed me, so I tapped my brakes really hard, and then the "fun" began.

As they changed lanes and came alongside of me, I glared at them like they were crazy and gave them the universal, shrugged shoulder, hands up, "What's your problem?" gesture. Apparently, this was not to their liking, as a handgun came out of the window and was pointed at my car. Luckily, I had a hot rod at the time, so I "punched it" and put my head down. They followed me, and several shots were fired, but they missed their mark and the young boys didn't catch up. I lost them in traffic, veered to the right at a fork in the road, and that was the end of it.

If I'd have had a better perspective of the situation and recognized that there was a fork in the road where I could've chosen to simply let it go in the beginning, none of that would've ever happened. I was extremely lucky…it could've ended much worse! To this day, when I pass people who've done stupid things in traffic, I don't even look at them. I pray for them and give them plenty of room. I've got a different, healthier perspective now that helps me see the fork in the road and avoid all kinds of issues *before* they happen.

GOOD RIPPLE EFFECTS

One often overlooked factor to consider in the big picture of your health is how your well-being affects those around you, both now and in the future. There are far-reaching ripple effects that may touch more people than you think. Through the years, working with a lot of patients has allowed me to see how the health of one individual can affect so many different other people.

Let's look at the positive side of things first. When you choose to seek good health, those in your circle of influence will be affected in a beneficial way. Your spouse and friends are more likely to be motivated to focus on their health when you show them an encouraging example. Having that focus also sets an example for your children and their friends who spend time at your home as to what is normal when it comes to being healthy. What you see your parents do often becomes what you do. Many adults are simply copying what their parents and sometimes even grandparents did.

I had a patient who became interested in health as he began to improve with chiropractic care and, eventually, the pain that had been plaguing him disappeared. He and I would discuss little health tips during each of his appointments, and then, one day, he made a decision to make another significant change in his health in addition to spinal alignment. He came from a family that was overweight and could be technically considered obese. I began to counsel him on diet and had the honor of encouraging him along the way with high fives and hugs as he lost weight and felt better.

His family began to notice and at first asked him if he was okay because he looked "a little too skinny." Then as he lost significant weight and approached a target weight based on his height and body frame, he began to get ridiculed and judged by them. They told him that he was crazy, unhealthy, trying to show off, and asked if he thought he was better than they were.

This weighed on his heart very heavily, but he maintained his goals and held firm. As time went by, they began to accept him as he continued to show them love and not fire back. As more time went by, they began to ask him how he did it, one by one. Now, over 10 years later, many of them have made tremendous changes in their health, lost a great deal of weight, and gained a wealth of energy and vitality. The truth is that he may have even saved some of their lives. Most of his family believed their genes had been to blame and they'd lost the genetic "lottery." However, this simply wasn't true. They had only to believe that they could make changes and then have an example to follow that was realistic for them.

The full ramifications of the choices we make will never be known completely in our lifetimes.

In the end, the ripple effects of him changing his life and improving his health may prove to affect countless thousands of people if you look down the road many years from now. The children, grandchildren, and great-grandchildren of his family members may have totally different futures based on this one man's decision to do something brave, challenging, and out of his comfort zone. He may have not even believed that he could lose weight, much less actually change the lives of his family and others for generations to come. Talk about ripple effects.

His story is an amazing one, and it only involves the diet component of the chemical pillar of the foundation of health. What if you were to make a decision about exercise or your attitude or your faith that affected generations to come? What if you set the example that played a role in the very direction of our nation or world because of your decision to improve your health? The full ramifications of the choices we make will never be known completely in our lifetimes.

Years ago, there was a missionary family who devoted their lives to loving, helping, and serving people in a third-world country. A young native boy latched on to them, helped them with whatever was needed, and traveled with them to all of the villages they went. He loved them and served them tirelessly. By some people's standards, they didn't accomplish much in that they couldn't really quantify how many—if any—people were really touched by their ministry. At best, their "success" would be considered average, both by them and by others.

They eventually became too old to do the kind of missions they'd been doing, so they retired and moved back to the United States, leaving behind the boy, who was now a young man. Eventually, they passed away without much fanfare and never had more than a mention about their life's mission ever get printed where anyone would even know that they existed.

The young boy who accompanied them, however, continued to learn and grow and mature. He went on to become one of the most influential and loved pastors in his country and touched the lives of hundreds of thousands of people. Without the humble missionary couple whose lives were examples of love, compassion, and grace, he almost certainly would've never become the man and leader he is today.

That faithful couple went on to heaven without ever knowing whether or not their ministry had amounted to anything, and may have even thought they'd failed. They could not have fathomed their legacy: They were indirectly responsible for a ministry that had ripple effects for generations to come. In the big picture, those ripples are undoubtedly still going, affecting millions of people today.

BAD RIPPLE EFFECTS

Unfortunately for all of us, how we live our lives can also have negative ripple effects for a long time as well. Routinely, I have patients who tell me how a fellow coworker was out sick and they were made to bear the burden, with long hours and work piled on their desk because of their coworker's absence. Now hold your horses—I realize that we all get sick, but some of us get sick way more often than we should because we don't take care of ourselves.

Tell the truth. How many times have you gotten sick after you stayed up too late, repeatedly, or were eating way too much junk food for a long period of time? On several occasions, I can tell you exactly what happened to me that created sickness in my life. One time in particular it was blatantly obvious to me why and how I got sick. It was as formulaic as a recipe for baking cookies. Put all the right ingredients together and you get a specific outcome. In this case, it was a bad recipe.

When my wife and I were dating, we decided to be youth leaders at a Young Life camp in the mountains. We were part of a group of around 80 kids and eight leaders. We set out from Orlando on a multi-bus road trip for about ten hours to the mountains. As you can imagine, these teenagers were goin' crazy and eating every kind of junk food imaginable. The bus ride was long—I mean, *really* long. My patience was tried to its extent, nerves were fried, and the strangulation of certain teens was strongly considered… frequently. (I'm only kidding; I only considered it once or twice.) ☺

We eventually made it to camp and managed to play hard the rest of the day, ate a meal consisting of white pasta, some thin red sauce, two slices of white bread, a square of mystery cake, and a tall glass of "fruit" punch. I'm pretty sure it was my pancreas that was getting fruit punched, trying to handle all of the carbs I had just ingested. Then, of course, the boys with whom I shared the cabin were full of vim and vigor and refused to sleep, no matter what was threatened. They finally collapsed from exhaustion, after a push-up contest at about four in the morning. I kid you not. Then, at six, right on cue, the bugle sounded and we were summoned to the mess hall for breakfast.

This "nutritious" meal consisted of pancakes, syrup, sugared cereal, donuts, and juice (and an insulin shot). The rest of the day was spent doing ridiculous but fun events of major physical exertion, dotted with more "meals" of processed carbs, and another late night. Exhaustion began to set in. This cycle continued for an entire week. Then, on the last night, it was in the lower 40's and there was a carnival night to celebrate the end of the camp. Kids voted to select which leaders would man the dunking booth. Guess who got nominated to be dunked? Yep. Me. Yay!

The water that filled the tank was from a snow melt-off creek and was barely above freezing. After being dunked for half an hour or so, over and over again, with the cold wind blowing on me, the party was finally over. It was time to load the buses for an all-night drive back home. As strange as it may sound, the kids didn't feel like going to sleep on the bus and wanted to yell, giggle, and annoy everyone around them until, oh, around five in the morning or so. I know! Weird, right? At six, we pulled into the parking lot back in Orlando. It was a life-changing camp for the kids and for us.

If there was ever a recipe for getting sick, I figured it out. The immune system can only handle so many insults until it fails and a person gets sick...and I did get sick, in grand fashion. Besides the fact that my life was affected by my choices, the lives of countless others were affected as well. Patients who were scheduled to come in were rescheduled, forced to endure discomfort for a longer period of time and disrupt their workweek at another time, perhaps an inconvenient one, to get back in to see me.

My girlfriend at the time, who is now my wife, also got sick, which imposed additional burdens on her coworkers. This hindered their ability to accomplish what they needed to do, resulting in extended hours that might have made them late to or even miss a kid's sports game or recital, causing a problem for a whole family. See what I'm getting at here? Ripple effects are powerful.

OTHER RIPPLE EFFECTS

Ripple effects of our health choices also change many other areas, like our health-care system, and then, by default, our taxes. When we, as a country, don't take care of our health, then there are many lost days of work, which hurts industry as well. When we're less healthy, get sick, and can't work, then businesses lose money due to lost productivity and we end up increasing the cost of health care. As people begin to fill up the hospitals as they age, they don't get to live the life they wanted, like traveling or spending time with family, and the cost of government-funded programs like Medicare and Medicaid go up. You then have to pay more taxes and spend a greater percentage of your income, leaving you less money to spend to stimulate the economy.

It's easy to say that in America we have the freedom to do whatever we want, but in many cases that means our choices affect someone else. As individuals and as a society, we benefit greatly from having a healthy population. We should begin incentivizing those who make good choices concerning their health and reach certain defined goals of weight, blood pressure, lean body mass index, and other lab work values.

People are willing to cut out a coupon to save a dollar on a package of food, but what if they could save hundreds of dollars every month on health-care premiums simply by becoming healthier? It wouldn't be punishing those who make poor choices but rewarding those who make good ones. If we're all supposed to "pull our weight" in health care, it sure makes sense that those who are less of a burden on the system should be required to pay less into it. Who's with me?

Sorry about the rant on health care and insurance, but as a doctor it's something that I deal with every day. Costs are skyrocketing and causing significant distress for people and their finances. However, there's good news for those of us who look to the Original Design for health and choose to make wise choices. Our personal health-care expenses will certainly be much less than those who make poor choices due to the fact that we simply don't have near the number of health issues to deal with! We can all make better choices.

A LACK OF HEALTH CAN BLOCK YOUR DESTINY

Another big-picture reason for living a healthy life is that you simply cannot accomplish in life what you were designed to when you're sick. I've touched on it multiple times before, but it bears repeating here: When you're unhealthy, you don't feel like doing much.

Have you ever noticed how, when you're sick and in bed, you barely have the energy to even read a book or pay a bill or make a sandwich? We're just plain useless when we're not feeling well. However, being unhealthy affects us much more than just when we're sick. When we're not firing on all cylinders, we miss out on so many opportunities throughout the day.

Many times, when we're even a little out of shape, we won't have the energy to keep the house clean, work on a project, or even play with the kids. Frankly, we're cheating our children out of the experiences with us which they yearn for. When a person is obese, or experiencing lung issues from smoking, just walking to the mailbox can be nearly impossible. Does that sound like the abundant health that we were designed to have?

When you have musculoskeletal pain from misalignments in your spine or other joints, it hurts to do the easiest of tasks, and many times compels you to skip them altogether. When you haven't been getting enough sleep, you are often too exhausted to accomplish even simple chores. When you're emotionally downtrodden, overburdened, overstressed, or depressed, you may even contemplate not going to work or spending time with friends and family. Can you see the trend here? You're being robbed of the quality of life that you were destined for.

If any one of the pillars of health are in bad shape, we can't fully experience what we were designed to do, or be who we were designed to be. If multiple pillars of the health's foundation are crumbling, then our very lives may be in jeopardy. Our poor choices concerning our health will not only affect us, but the ripple effects will affect our entire world around us. Luckily for us, however, our bodies were designed so that they can be mistreated, and yet, with good choices over time, they can often regain their structure and function, and we can reclaim the lives we were designed to live.

**Fulfillment in life is much simpler than that—
to be in constant awe and appreciation of the beauty
of all you've been given, choosing to ignore the
negative feelings associated with what you were not.**

IN THE END

In the end, what exactly are we all really looking for in the big picture of life? If you ask most people, and force them to narrow down their answer to one or two words, they would say something like love, God, peace, happiness, meaning, purpose, fulfillment, or health. Sadly, it's way too often that people are striving to achieve, under their own power, things that will never satisfy. We've been trained to believe that pushing harder and working more is a good thing, and it can be to a point, but it's more about what you're working *for*.

This reminds me of the story of Howard Hughes, the self-made multimillionaire who, in the end of his life, was asked what would make him happy. He said, "One more dollar." He later lost his mind and died. Sad story, but it's true. So many things we're led to believe will make us happy, like money, fame, possessions, and power, are actually hollow, pointless pursuits. In the end, they tend to create destruction and despair, not health and happiness. Fulfillment in life is much simpler than that—to be in constant awe and appreciation of the beauty of all you've been given, choosing to ignore the negative feelings associated with what you were not.

Several years ago I had a half dozen weekends where I was away from home due to meetings, conferences, and other trips. I missed my wife and girls terribly. On the last of those Saturdays, I got up early and was backing out of the garage when my oldest daughter, Audrey, came running out of the house. She was crying and pleading with me, "Daddy, please don't go! Please don't leave me *again*!" I told her very sweetly that I had to attend this conference and that I'd see her in a few days. I pulled out of the driveway with her still crying and begging for me to stay.

That moment was a fork in the road for me where I needed to get some perspective and look at the big picture. I stopped at the end of the street and thought about it for a second. If I died that day, would the conference or time with my daughter be more important? Of course, it was no contest and I turned around and pulled into the driveway with her still sitting on the front porch with Mommy holding and consoling her as she sobbed. When she saw me, her face lit up, she ran to me, and we both began to cry tears of joy. We had an awesome weekend together as a family.

As I and many others have said before, life is a journey, not a destination. Enjoy the ride. Should we strive to improve ourselves and achieve more in life? Of course, but let's remember to be grateful for each day, each smile, each flower, each minute, and what we already have in front of us. In the end, living with a heart of thanks for where we are and what we have will put out the fire of discontentedness for where we aren't and what we don't have. An attitude of gratitude will absolutely destroy sadness, anger, envy, frustration, and depression.

Let's try to remember to regularly take a step back and look at the big picture. We've got to be a part of something bigger than ourselves. All—not only a few—of the things we've discussed in the previous chapters have a powerful effect on our health and the health of those around us. If we adhere to the Original Design for health as the foundation for our lives, we will find health, happiness, love, and purpose. We'll see so many good things fall into place, not just for us but for our families, our communities, our nations, and our whole planet.

CHAPTER 17

THE 3 EASY STEPS

So, how do you get started? If you feel overwhelmed, or like there's a whole list of areas that you'd like to change but can't seem to figure out how to take the first step, let me help. As we've gone through this book, we've touched on so many areas of health, but don't worry. You don't need to change them all at once. Hopefully you've learned something, you've been inspired, and you feel ready to make at least a little change in your life.

When you boil it all down, after you've done some self-education, it's time to take the three easy steps that begin the process of change. I know these steps seem simple, but less than 10% of people who set out to accomplish something actually implement these three steps. Don't be one of those people. Make the decision right now to do something different and follow through with what you've learned. This is where it starts, not where it ends.

Being totally honest with yourself opens the door to real and permanent change.

STEP 1: ANALYZE WHERE YOU ARE RIGHT NOW

If you remember back in the Introduction, I talked about how all of the pillars are equally important. You'll be tempted to work on just one or two because you think that they're more important than the others. But I'm telling you that you cannot separate any of them out as being more critical than any other one in creating overall health. They're all important in forming an ideal balance and optimal health according to the Original Design.

It's finally time to do an analysis, take an inventory of where you are, and make a list of things to change in all the pillars of health. You have to be totally and brutally honest with yourself here. Minimizing a problem or shortfall is only going to hurt you and slow your progress. Let it all out. You know what you're not doing right, where you're coming up short, and what you're unhappy with. You may have even discovered a few new areas that you need to change.

If you don't want anyone else to see what you're writing, then by all means keep your list private. It's for you and *your* personal health, after all, and not for anyone else. Because you're unique, there's no value in only doing what someone else does; ask God to help you see where you need to change. You can be the healthiest you've ever been. Don't worry about what others around you are doing; for once in your life, this is all about you.

Again, don't hold back or try to make your list look better than it really is. That's not going to help you. Living in denial is one of the greatest barriers to achieving true change. Being totally honest with yourself opens the door to real and permanent change.

**All great accomplishments begin with a great plan,
and all great plans begin with a great dream.**

STEP 2: CREATE NEW GOALS AND A PLAN

As you look at your analysis of each of the areas of health, feel free to reference this book and other sound advice in the Resources section, and write down what you want to achieve according to the suggestions for goal setting below. Many books on goal setting tell you to have short-, mid- and long-term goals. You might even get as detailed as goals for the day, week, and month, or for the season, the year, every ten years, and so on. This is a great idea, but even if you lump all your goals all together, it's a great start—it'll just take longer to check off the long-term goals. Think baby steps here. Even writing down a few goals will make a big difference.

Maybe you've realized that you're actually only getting six and a half hours of sleep when you know you really need eight hours. You might decide that the appropriate steps would be to have a short-term goal of getting an extra 30 minutes of sleep over the next month. Your midterm goal might be to bump that number up to one hour over the following six months. Finally, your long-term goal might be to commit to bumping it up to a full eight hours of sleep from that point forward.

Start off with small goals. The idea behind this is that it's easier to do a little bit at a time than it is to try and get an additional hour and a half of sleep immediately when you haven't done that in years. Try to be realistic, but don't hold back. Life is short and we only get one shot at this. Should you set up crazy big goals too? Absolutely. All great accomplishments begin with a great plan, and all great plans begin with a great dream. Dream big! If you don't dream big, you won't achieve big.

**Writing down goals for each pillar of health
is absolutely crucial to your success.**

Setting goals is critical to success in every area of your life. I've heard it said that living life without goals is like playing basketball without a hoop. How would you know what to aim for, and how would you keep score?

An important ingredient in making successful goals is to be as specific as possible. The more specific you are with your goal, the more you've thought about it, and the more likely you are to achieve it. You want to develop your goals with as many details as possible. Describe the goal with all five of your senses. Consider what it will look like—its color, size, shape, etc. Think about what it will be like to touch it, taste it, smell it, and how it will make you feel when it's realized.

One other piece of advice that is critical in achieving goals is to write them down. This has been discussed so many times in self-help books that it nearly goes without saying, and yet so many people don't do it. They may say they write their goals down, but they can't actually produce a piece of paper or a digital file with them written down. There's something magical that happens in your brain and heart when you crystalize what you're thinking about and take it from the mental realm to the physical realm by writing it down. It's been proven over and over again.

Writing down goals for each pillar of health is absolutely crucial to your success. Here's an example of a simple chart you can copy onto a notepad, or print off of my website to make your own. Create a page (or multiple if necessary) of goals for each of the four pillars of health: emotional, physical, chemical, and spiritual.

GOAL	TERM	ACTION STEPS
1. Read The Original Design for Health	one month	Divide the number of pages by 31 and read that many pages per day.
2. Eat healthier	one week	Skip soda in the afternoon and have water with lemon and stevia instead.
3.		

STEP 3: START WITH ONE THING AT A TIME

All of life's journeys begin with one step. I remember when I started writing this book. I'd been thinking about it and even compiling information for nearly 20 years. One summer night in 2008, while in California to work with Andy Roddick at a tennis tournament for a few days, I sat in a hotel room staring at an empty Word document and a blinking cursor. That's where it all began. All I had was the idea, a passion to share it and the desire to write about it.

Needless to say, I felt extremely overwhelmed. I had no idea where to start. So I began doubting myself and whether or not I had any business writing a book. I heard the voices of people in my head who had shot me down and laughed at my goal, some of whom were close to me. What did I do? I started with a prayer. I asked God to guide me and give me the words and courage and strength to write this book. I then wrote the first two words: Original Design. It had begun with one simple step—a title. Then I wrote the next three words: In the beginning. I had taken another small step. One step at a time, with God's guidance, an idea, a plan, and a belief that I could do it, and I began to write…even if only a few lines.

At times the steps were easy and words flowed like Niagara Falls. Other days were tough, there was barely a trickle, and I wanted to give up. I trusted that it would all work out and I did what I could. I continued to take small steps. And over eight years later, the book is sitting on the shelves of Barnes & Noble.

Listen, your goals don't just happen. You have to start taking steps in the right direction. I may not know how to walk from my house to the beach, but I do know that I need to face south and I know that I have to take steps—so that's where I'll start. I'll simply do what I *know* to do and figure it out from there.

With diet, you might decide to simply start with trading your unhealthy snacks for healthy ones. Maybe you decide to cut out eating junky, processed carbs when you're at home and be in better control of your choices. You could start by adding one or two servings of organic fruits and vegetables where you had never done that before. Those are all great starts. They are by no means a stopping point but a jumping off point to begin your health transformation.

It might be slow at first, but then one day you'll look back and be blown away by the difference in your life.

When I first started in chiropractic, I had a patient who came in for nutritional counseling and we went through all kinds of consulting, analysis, and training. I was great! I mean, I really gave her some great info and quite dynamically, I might add—or so I thought. At the end of it all she said, "Thank you! That was great information. I actually learned a lot, but… uh…there's no way I'm doing that." I was stunned. They didn't prepare me in school for a patient that doesn't want to do what I'm suggesting. I said a quick prayer in my heart, and then these words came out: "Well, okay, umm…what would you normally have for dinner tonight?" She said, "Oh, well, it's Tuesday and we go to a Mexican restaurant that has a "Two-fer Tuesday" deal. You get two margaritas, two plates of enchiladas, and two desserts for the price of one."

I said, "Cool. So go there and order everything you'd normally order." She looked stunned and said, "I *like* this diet." Then I added, "But just eat half—half the margarita, half the chips and salsa, half the enchiladas, and half the dessert. You'll have leftovers!" She squeaked out a timid "I think I can do that." In six months, she lost over 50 pounds, and then said, "Okay, will you tell me about broccoli again?"

Initially, she wasn't willing to tackle all of the changes, so we just started with *one* step—how much she was eating. From there she was ready to take on more and more change and began to eat much more healthily. She eventually lost over 100 pounds! She wasn't making any better choices about the quality of her food, only the quantity of it. However, with time she felt better all-around and began making many different positive choices for her health, including the quality of food that she ate, exercise and rest. She loved what she saw in the mirror and how she felt.

It wasn't just the weight loss, though, that transformed her life. Her immune system improved, she had a ton more energy, her joints stopped hurting, she got off all of her medications, she did more things with friends and family, and her self-esteem and emotional health skyrocketed. She bought new clothes, smiled more, and even began to wear makeup. Each of the intertwined benefits of becoming healthy moved her closer and closer to the person she was originally designed to be. And it all started with one step.

It might be slow at first, but then one day you'll look back and be blown away by the difference in your life. It's hard in the beginning, but repetition creates a pattern, and over time a pattern becomes a habit. And as they say, habits are hard to break. That's a good thing when it's a good habit. You'll see that this is now the new you. You'll undoubtedly have discovered many areas that you need to change. So, again, don't let this be overwhelming. Just start with one simple step, something you know you can do. You can't change everything today and you don't need to.

As you continue your journey of learning, you'll more fully understand an area of health and be more motivated and confident in changing what you're currently doing. Then, step by step, you'll find yourself happier, healthier, and becoming exactly who God originally designed you to be.

NEVER STOP LEARNING

Part of the message I want to get across to people is that they should never stop learning. There's no way that I or any other health professional can pass along all of the information that we have in our brains, which we've learned over dozens of years on our own personal and professional journeys. It's up to you to continue your journey too.

It's pivotal that you understand that you must take responsibility for your own health. There's something that has become extremely clear to me as I have studied nutrition and health, and been around it for over 40 years. It's that the more people rely on TV, radio, magazine or internet articles as the sole source for information on how to stay healthy, the more likely they are to fall prey to some short-sighted business ploy or personal agenda.

The bottom line is that most of the information that you read or hear is aimed at selling you something for their benefit, not yours. You'll get really bad information that leads to misguided beliefs and the wrong plan that's based on ever-changing opinions and trends. The Original Design for health, however, is the same yesterday, today, and forever.

As most of you have already figured out, there's a ton of information on the subject of health. So how does one sort through all of it? The majority of people have to sift through all the information themselves, but that's why I wrote *The Original Design for Health* in the first place. This book was birthed from my heart's desire to simplify a challenging concept: How do we achieve our greatest level of health? That's a tall order, but hopefully this book has made it a little easier to understand the bigger picture.

On a daily basis in my chiropractic practice, I field questions from people who "heard this or read that" and don't know how to discern fact from fiction, or a straight-up scam. That's why at the beginning of this book I mentioned one of the guiding principles of the Original Design, which is that it should be simple, easy to understand, easy to do, and be based on tried-and-true practices and ideas that just make good sense and have stood the test of time.

I've always appreciated some wise statements that Thomas Edison made in 1902. They seem to fit the growing trend of modern health practitioners today to educate their patients on how to stay healthy. He said, "Medicine is played out...The doctor of the future will give no medicine, but will instruct his patient in the care of the human frame, in diet and in the cause and prevention of diseases." He went on to say that all the scientific discoveries were "tending to the simple truth—that you can't improve on nature." I don't know about you, but to me, that kinda sounds like what I've been talking about. He could see that there was a pre-existing Original Design that needed to be the focus for a proactive approach to health in the future.[1]

In the Resources section that follows, you have a list of "doctors of the future," organizations, books, websites, authors, and pastors who offer great information to continue your learning journey. They may differ on some specifics, and maybe even a few core principles, but overall they're all solid sources of information. We're all unique individuals, so slightly different plans to achieve optimal health are to be expected, as long as they adhere to the Original Design.

It's up to you now. Educate yourself a little more each day and delve deeper into subjects as you have interest or need. You'll be able to glean *something* good from everything you take in, even if you can't agree with everything they say. Remember: Knowledge is power, and the application of that knowledge is wisdom. Whether it's for yourself or someone you love, I encourage you to continue your education on health in such a way that it'll arm you with the information you need to live your life the way it was intended to be lived, according to *The Original Design for Health.*

TURBO NUTSHELL
QUICK-START SYNOPSIS

Soooo…you're one of *those* people, huh? You're the kind of person who reads the end of the book first to find out what happens. Mmmhmm. I know who you are. That's because I'm one of those people and it's why I put this section in the book. Some might say that you have ADD, but I'd just say that you have a desire to be efficient with your time. What you're about to read are the main principles and absolute core of what this book is all about.

The problem with a synopsis is that so much of understanding something is learning the background information that goes along with it. It's a little like hearing somebody's comments out of context. It'll make a whole lot more sense and give you way more confidence and resolve for making changes in your life if you read the whole book. Let me strongly urge you to go back to Chapter 1, pace yourself, and make a plan to challenge yourself to read a little bit each day or each week to fully understand what I'm trying to say, how this all works, and how you'll benefit from applying what you read. But if you insist on skipping ahead, it's turbo fast, wrapped up in a nutshell, and will get you started quickly. Here we go.

Introduction

I'm a second-generation chiropractor and nutritionist and have spent my whole life around health care. I feel like I've been called to share with the world an idea that refocuses our complicated and disjointed approach to living a healthy and happy life to a simple, easily understandable and logical one. I want to uncomplicate things and make it easy for anyone to do.

The idea is that God had a plan, and still has a plan, for everything in this world, including our health. I call this the Original Design. The closer we adhere to that plan, the healthier we'll be. And the further we stray from that plan, the greater our individual and collective health problems will be. In fact, we're in a major decline in health in industrialized societies today. We're advancing in health and science technology, and yet we're getting sicker by the day.

We all know that there are multiple factors that affect our levels of health, like sleep, nutrition, and exercise. There are four pillars of health that all of these factors can be grouped into: mental, physical, chemical, and spiritual pillars of the foundation of health. In order to reach optimal health, our goal is to keep the pillars of the foundation equal and balanced, the way it was designed to be in the beginning.

Chapter 1: In the Beginning...

In the beginning, God created everything in the universe, including humans and a plan for them to be healthy. Ninety percent of humans on earth believe that there is a God. It's logical to me that if God exists, then He designed a perfect plan for the world and everything in it to work in a certain way. He would've paid attention to every detail.

Nearly everything that you see in this world or use in your life has a specific purpose, and when used in the correct way it's the most effective and valuable. Design just makes sense. For instance, you might be able to slowly hammer in a nail with a screwdriver, but that screwdriver was not designed to put in nails. When you use it as a hammer, it's weak and ineffective. However, when you use it for what it was designed to do, it works extremely well. It's all part of the Original Design for that tool. Likewise, we are the happiest, healthiest, and feel the most fulfilled when we're doing what we were designed to do.

However, when we veer from the Original Design, it can create (and has already created) uncountable issues for the human race and the planet as a whole, which can have anywhere from small to massive consequences. The good news is that even though we seem to be really good at messing everything up, we're also capable of changing and regaining what we've lost, at least to a great degree. We can achieve higher levels of health by refocusing our hearts, minds, and bodies on the Original Design.

Chapter 2: Balance

As we touched on earlier in the Introduction, balancing the pillars of health should be our primary focus if we're truly interested in living at the highest level of health. Most of us realize that we're the happiest and healthiest when we're feeling well, making a good living, and in loving relationships, etc. We feel balanced.

One of the guiding principles of this book is found in looking at plants. From early on, we're all taught that a plant needs four basic requirements: water, sunlight, air, and soil. The exact amounts and kinds may differ based on the type of plant, but the four *basic* requirements remain the same for all plants and each are equally important: You can't give a plant the perfect soil, clean air, and the perfect amount of light, but never water it. Each of the needs of the plant must be met and kept in balance to have a happy, healthy plant.

The question of course is, how do we create balance in our lives? It's not a simple answer, but it's not rocket science either. It's a process by which we look at all of the areas of our lives that affect our health and decide which of those factors need some change. Then we create a plan for change and implement it in order to create balance and a greater level of health.

PILLAR I: MENTAL

Chapter 3: Perception and Attitude

As most of us know and have personally experienced, the way two people view any given event and what they perceive can vary widely. They might have experienced the exact same event, but they each will tell two different stories and would be able to pass a lie-detector test to verify that they truly believe their "side of the story." How we perceive anything is based on a number of factors, like upbringing, religious beliefs, past experiences, and our emotional state at the time. We need to shape our perception of the world around us based on as much fact and good information from God's Word and time-tested examples as possible. We only have to be careful about who and what we trust.

Attitude determines so much of how we live our lives and how we feel—mentally, physically, and spiritually. Contrary to what some believe, we all *choose* to have a good or a bad attitude. Most of us live our lives as if our emotions and attitudes were a leaf in a hurricane, totally at the mercy of the wind. It doesn't have to be that way, and you can change that helpless, reactionary type of lifestyle.

There's a statement that I share with patients, friends, and family almost every day: "It's not the circumstances of life that determine our level of peace, health, and happiness, but the attitude with which we endure them." We were designed to overcome the circumstances that surround us, *not* to live with a victim mentality.

Chapter 4: Emotions

Emotion is extremely powerful and is usually a direct result of the events of our lives that we have already experienced and what we're worrying about in the future. We can't measure our emotional health level with a lab test, but I came up with a quick and simple test to get a rough idea of where you're at emotionally. Be sure to take the test for a quick check-up.

All of us are motivated by two things: fear or reward. Either of those motivational factors involve our emotions in that we're either trying to avoid something or trying to get something. Most of us are dealing with something that affects how we think, act, and speak. Nearly all of us have had in the past or are currently experiencing issues that are adversely affecting us. These hurts typically involve someone we need to forgive and emotions that we need to let go of.

Emotions are intangible, but their effect on us is very tangible. For instance, someone tells you that you're fat, and that hurts you. You can't see or measure that emotional damage, but you then might eat more food because of the resulting emotional stress. Then, you can measure the physical effects, like an expanding waistline, that change as a result. Intangible emotions cause tangible actions.

To sum it all up, emotions are quite real and greatly affect how we act and feel. We have to isolate the negative emotions in our lives, determine where they're coming from, and then eliminate them. At the same time, we have to identify positive emotions and focus on them as a source of happiness to attain the optimal health we were designed to live.

Chapter 5: Reality and Change

When you start reading a book about health, you can often get excited about making changes, but then reality sets in and you realize that it's hard. That's okay. It's not about being perfect or changing everything all at once; it's about making small changes as you can, and slowly working toward bigger goals.

As you're evaluating all the areas of your life that affect your health, you have to make some tough decisions about whether or not something is good for you. To do this, you can determine the Net Health Effect (NHE) of something to help you determine its value. For example, jogging seems like a healthy choice, but if you do it on concrete, down the side of the interstate, in beat-up ole sneakers, in 105-degree heat, with bad posture, while inhaling exhaust fumes and enduring all the pounding of the joints of the feet, ankles, knees, hips, and spine, its NHE would be negative. Pick things that have a positive NHE and you're off to a good start.

After you decide what needs to change, the time to face reality and make the change is right now! Make the changes before the damage occurs. This could be about anything in your life, from diet to a relationship that has strayed from the Original Design and negatively affects you. Your ideal health and all of the factors that affect it are unique to you. You can't follow someone else's Original Design. Remember, you *can* change and you might just be the healthiest that you've ever been.

Chapter 6: Relationships

Relationships are central to human life and provide amazing health benefits in so many different ways. They give us someone to share the good times and the bad times with, and they are truly critical to the healthy human experience. If we aren't in relationship with others, we can get weird and miss out on the richness of life that we were designed to experience.

Our relationship with God is of primary importance, and then the relationship with our spouse (if you're married). Keeping our marriage alive and healthy is important to our state of well-being, as well as that of our children's. You have to work on it and never stop dating your spouse. If we want our spouses to look at us like they did back when we were dating, then we have to do what we did and be who we were back then.

If you're only dating, then make sure that you fully envision who it is you want to be with and don't compromise and choose someone who is close *but* has a long list of issues. We're not talking about minor issues here, but about big issues that can really wreck your health. Those "buts" can truly come back and bite you in the end (see what I did there?). Never date people with "big buts."

Choose your friends carefully, because they can have big "buts" too. It's often been said that you end up like the people you hang around. That's true—I've seen it so often with friends in my own life and patients at the office. Also, find a mentor or two who can help shape you into the person you feel like you're supposed to be. Surround yourself with relationships that encourage and inspire you; they'll help you become who you were designed to be.

Chapter 7: Playtime

What could be more fun than playtime? We all love to play, but we all tend to like different ways of doing it. We all enjoy different things because we were all designed to do different things with our lives. When we do the things that really get us charged up, then we're activating a unique system that God has placed within us.

Our bodies produce all kinds of chemicals, hormones, and neurotransmitters associated with experiencing pleasure. During playtime, a dopamine response from the adrenal glands stimulates the natural reward circuitry of our brains, giving us intense emotions relating to love, excitement, fun, happiness, peace, pleasure, and laughter. That's playtime.

In following the things that you enjoy and excel at, you're producing this dopamine response, and by experiencing fun, you're engaging the mechanism that God designed for you to discover who you were designed to be. However, some people have their priorities out of whack and feel like they're too tired to play. That's no good. We have to take out time for recreation. In fact, if you break down that word, it's "re-" and "creation." Playtime isn't only a mental vacation; it helps you to re-create who you were designed to be and to help you find your purpose. Make it a priority.

PILLAR II: PHYSICAL

Chapter 8: Alignment

As a chiropractor, I believe that alignment is absolutely critical to one's overall health. I've been around it my whole life and have experienced it personally, as well as with my patients, for more than 20 years. It's so simple. Your body has an underlying framework like a house or a car. When that framework is aligned correctly, according to its Original Design, it will work properly and won't cause you pain or dysfunction. Conversely, when it's out of its proper alignment, there will be some combination of pain, muscle spasm, inflammation, altered sensation, and dysfunction…or all of the above. The symptom is the cue that there's an underlying root problem.

The other part of this equation that not everybody knows is that organ and muscle function can be related to spinal alignment. For instance, neurologists will ask their patients with severe low back pain and a suspected herniated disc, that's causing tingling and numbness down the leg, if they've experienced any loss in control of their bowel or bladder. This is because nerve irritation in the lower lumbar spine can be the cause.

In addition to the spine, all joints, including elbows, wrists, knees, and shoulders, are commonly misaligned and can create dysfunction like carpal tunnel, plantar fasciitis, and tennis elbow. This is why Olympic and professional level athletes seek out our help, but truly everyone on the planet can benefit from chiropractic care. Trying to live a healthy life, free of pain, and functioning to your maximum capacity is best achieved by having your body realigned or adjusted to as close to its Original Design as possible.

Chapter 9: Exercise

All right, I know, I know. Most of you hate exercise. But when you think about it, haven't there been times in your life where you've been sweatin' like a pig, burnin' calories like crazy, and you didn't even realize that you were exercising? Having fun is the secret to great exercise that will make it easy for you to keep it a consistent habit in your life. It has a lot to do with your state of mind. It doesn't really matter what you do.

It's really important to do *something*, though. Find ways to incorporate exercise in your daily life, at your desk, or while you're driving or watching TV. It's easy—you only have to make up your mind to do it. Motion is the key to joint health. Exercise has so many positive effects on your health, affecting nearly all of the other aspects of health. It has a beneficial influence on energy, sleep, depression, pain relief, self-esteem, strength, blood pressure, stability, stress, cleansing, weight control, mental clarity, spiritual health, and much more.

While I don't tell people what kind to do, I do suggest doing exercises that are low impact and work the front and the back, the left side and the right side, and the top and the bottom of all of your muscle groups. The more muscle groups that you maintain, the better off you'll be and the closer you'll stay to your Original Design.

You want to stay active and healthy, and that means taking it easy on your body while still keeping everything moving. Therefore, stretching is also important to do throughout the day to keep fluids pumping, to keep joints from locking up, and to keep muscles from getting too tight. Exercise and stretching help keep our bodies in the shape that they were originally designed to be in so we can do the things we were designed to do and be who we were designed to be.

Chapter 10: Rest

This is an area of health that most of us know we're deficient in. Rest could be defined as any period of time at which your body is completely at ease and you're allowing your body and mind to relax. It could be sitting on a park bench and relaxing or listening to music while kicking back on the couch, or it could be getting a good night's sleep.

The average adult needs to get eight hours of sleep each night, but people usually know if they do okay on seven, or if they actually need nine to function and feel their best. This requirement changes based on many factors, including activity level and whether or not you're fighting an illness. There's a great chart to see how much we need at different ages in life. I have discovered, since my wife and I brought children into this world, that sleep is something that plays a critical role in determining how I feel and function, both mentally and physically. It's also an area of health that has a significant role in the function of our immune system and emotional health.

Napping is something I highly recommend to my patients, my own staff members, and anyone else who'll listen. Every day I take a 20-minute nap and suggest that getting between 15 and 30 minutes daily can drastically change your energy and immune level throughout the day. After lunch is usually best. Research has shown that taking a nap significantly increases your productivity and focus in the second half of the day and boosts your immune system. Einstein and Edison believed in naps, too!

If God rested on the seventh day and designed you to get sleepy every night, it's clearly part of the Original Design that you stay caught up on sleep and stay well rested. Rest is critical to your overall health.

PILLAR III: CHEMICAL

Chapter 11: Diet

Well, if this isn't the single most controversial topic in health, then I don't know what is. There's always someone telling us what to eat and what not to eat. There are books about diets of every kind that frequently tout ideas that are in complete opposition with each other. One diet says that you need to stay away from meat and avoid it like the plague, while the other says that you need to stuff a sausage with steak, wrap it in bacon, and eat it with gravy made from fat drippings.

Interestingly, the only thing that most experts agree on is that we need to stop eating processed fake foods, and eat more fresh (and I would add that they be organic) vegetables and fruit. The greatest amount of disagreement seems to involve protein and carbs. If you look around you, it becomes quickly apparent that while we all have an Original Design, that design is different and unique for each one of us.

It's my opinion that it's extremely ridiculous, cavalier, delusional, illogical, and irrational to suggest that there is one diet that is ideal for all of us. If we forget all of the opinions of the so-called experts, and our friend at work and our aunt Margaret who just read something in a magazine, we've done ourselves a huge favor and we're at a good starting point.

With our slate clean, what foods do we suppose we were originally designed to eat? Whole, organic, unprocessed real foods like vegetables, fruits, wild-caught fish, pastured meats, dairy and eggs, sprouted grains, nuts, clean water, and otherwise foods that were put on this earth by God to be eaten. It's designed to be simple. However, for every bit of damage that harsh processing, genetic engineering, chemical additives, hormones or any other alteration to the Original Design Diet that's done, the further from health and the closer to illness we will be.

Chapter 12: Supplements

Like diet, there are a wide variety of opinions about what supplements you should take. Supplements are big business and are often partial or total junk. Every company tells you that their supplements are the best and they'll have a whole line of different concoctions that will "cure what ails you." People regularly come to me who've joined a multilevel marketing company, and now, in addition to their day job, they tell me about their new occupation as a "nutritional consultant" and hand me a business card to that effect. Then they explain how I can "get rich quick" by selling the "miracle cure." Sound likely? Nope, not to me either.

I do believe in supplementation, though, because, as a matter of convenience, it's a way for busy people living in the modern world to get some of the nutrients they're missing in the Standard American Diet (SAD). My suggestion is to aim for securing the majority of your nutrition from your diet outlined in the diet section, and then use the help of a nutritionist to determine what you might be missing, how much of it you need, and how long you should take it.

As for picking a supplement company, I'd suggest one that uses organic whole foods as their raw products source, and only removes moisture and fiber to make their supplements. The vast majority of the supplements on the shelves today are from synthetic sources and you have no idea as to their origin, potency, or their bioavailability. They're incomplete and lack enzymes and other cofactors that make them as functional in the human body as naturally occurring vitamins. Supplements should be as close as possible to the Original Design of the foods they're made from in order to be useful and not harmful.

PILLAR IV: SPIRITUAL

Chapter 13: Intelligent Design

I would be remiss if I didn't discuss ID in this book because it has some obvious parallels to the Original Design. Learning about ID helps us understand that we and every living thing on our planet are not just a random accident, but are, in fact, intricately and amazingly designed. For many, knowing where we came from is the foundation of their faith.

To explain the existence of life on earth, you first have to account for the origin of the essential building blocks for every living cell on earth, which are large complex molecules called proteins. Proteins are created with the use of blueprints or instructions called DNA that guide the entire process. The amount of information in human DNA alone is roughly equivalent to 12 sets of encyclopedias, which equals 384 volumes' worth of detailed information that would fill 48 feet of library shelves.

These DNA instructions allow for the creation of every living cell in your body. How do we know they didn't happen by sheer accident? It's simple. Every day scientists use common sense to differentiate between random naturally occurring things and obviously intelligently designed things, and so do we. If you see the faces of past presidents on Mount Rushmore, for example, do you assume that they were made by wind and erosion? Of course not! There simply are no accidental natural causes that could create this kind of formation. That's common-sense science.

Only intelligent designers make meaningful and easily recognizable patterns or designs that scientists call information. If we conclude that there is an intelligent designer who created DNA and the information inside of it, then we can look into nature and expect to find order and beauty and design in all living things. Man, do we! We see it all around us, and it's truly amazing.

In knowing that there's an intelligent design and blueprints for even the smallest of molecules, it solidifies in my heart that there was and is an Original Design for everything, including little ole me. For me, that settles the idea of the existence of a Creator once and for all. I know that I'm not a random accident but I have a purposeful design—and *that* changes everything. If I just refer to the Original Design, then I can get my health back on track. This knowledge strengthens my spiritual health and therefore improves my overall health.

Chapter 14: Faith

This subject is one of those subjects that people are understandably extremely opinionated about, and it's not to be discussed quickly or lightly. I highly recommend reading this chapter in detail, but if you really want a short version, here goes…

Faith, as defined in this chapter, is a broad category that encompasses all of the aspects of one's beliefs and ideas surrounding the existence of God. Again, according to research, approximately 90% of the population of the planet believes in God or a Creator in some form or another. To me, without belief in God, the concept of health would have no point. If you don't believe in God and you're a random accident on a whirling rock in space, then what value could you possibly have for your life?

Since the vast majority of us believe in God, however, then we are mostly on the same page. There's no way that I'm going to suggest that we all believe the same thing, as you can't usually get two people in the same church to agree on everything. We all believe something; it's just a matter of what we believe.

At the heart of a conversation about God is the search for love, which is the most powerful force in the universe. You can see the effects of love now and throughout history, but you can't see it or touch it or measure it or prove it. We're taught that God is love, and so, in much the same way that you can't prove that love exists, you can't prove that God exists. We all search for significance and meaning and wonder where we came from. In seeking answers about your faith, you will find them…and God will find you.

CONCLUSION

Chapter 15: Input/Output

You often hear that computers are input/output machines, meaning that whatever you put into the computer is what's available to come out. The *only* thing, in fact, that can come out of it is what was put into it. In other words, if you don't first put something in, then you can't get anything out. We're much like a computer in that we can't think or talk or act the way we should unless we first have that information inside of us. However, while what has happened to you in the past may be something that you can't forget, it certainly doesn't determine what you'll do, what you'll say, or who you'll be in the future. Only you can decide that.

For instance, let's go back to the old phrase we heard when we were kids: "You are what you eat." Most of us would agree that it's true to a great extent. If you eat junk food, your body is going to become junky, and you'll begin to gain weight, have sickness, and experience dysfunction and pain. This is no accident. However, if you put the right food in your body, there's a much greater chance that you're going to have good health, normal function, very little pain, and a much more enjoyable life. Your greatest level of health can be ahead of you!

Very soon you could have the most physical health, emotional stability, spiritual strength, peace, and joy in your life that you've ever had by changing what you put inside of your mind, body, heart, and soul. Starting today, begin your journey with just one little step. When you do, you'll be able to take two steps tomorrow, and so on. It won't be an overnight transformation, but it'll be faster than you think.

We simply have to deliberately input information into our brains' database which helps us grow and believe in positive ways, and steers our output toward our Original Design.

Chapter 16: The Big Picture

There are so many times when I wish that I could have some kind of a reset button that would instantly give me the appropriate perspective and remind me of just how blessed I am. This magical button would remind me of how privileged I am to live in the country that I live in, and to have all the freedoms that I have. I'd be able to see the big picture and be completely aware of the value of my family, my friends, my ability to worship freely, to practice my profession, to own my home, and the opportunity I have to create my own destiny.

I think one good thing to do on a daily basis to get a big-picture perspective is to start off every day with prayer. I'll often pray that God allows me to see the forks in the road of life. Which fork we choose will have massive implications in the direction our lives take. At many points throughout a day, we all have an opportunity to choose one of several actions, responses, or attitudes concerning nearly anything in life. The powerful choice is to pray for the perspective that allows you to recognize the fork in the road before it actually happens.

One thing to consider in the big picture of your health that some people often overlook is how your health affects those around you, both now and in the future. There are far-reaching ripple effects that may be either good or bad, and are affecting more people than you think. Working with a lot of patients through the years has allowed me to see how the health of one individual can affect so many different other people. We want to make healthy choices in our lives that also positively affect the health of those around us.

In the end, what exactly is it that we're all really looking for in the big picture of life? Most people would say something like health, happiness, love, or purpose. If we stick close to the Original Design for health as the foundation for our lives, then we'll find what we're looking for and see so many good things fall into place for not only us, but our families, our communities, our nations, and our whole planet.

Chapter 17: The 3 Easy Steps

Sorry, you don't get a shortcut for this one. Come on, you can do it. It's not that long and it is pretty to the point anyway. Besides, after reading the turbo nutshell synopsis of all the other chapters, aren't you inspired to go back and read the whole thing anyway? I promise you'll love it. More good stuff awaits. Stay hungry, my friends.

NOTES

INTRODUCTION

1. National Center for Health Statistics, "Deaths: Final Data for 2013," Number of Deaths by 113 Selected Causes Table 10, by Jiquan Xu, et al., http://www.cdc.gov/nchs/data/nvsr/nvsr64/nvsr64_02.pdf.

2. Barbara Starfield, MD, MPH, "Is US Health Really the Best in the World?" *Journal of the American Medical Association* 284, no. 4 (2000): 483–485.

3. National Center for Health Statistics, *Health, United States, 2015*, Obesity Among Children and Adolescents Table 59, http://www.cdc.gov/nchs/data/hus/hus15.pdf.

4. S. Swan, et al., "Have Sperm Densities Declined? A Re-analysis of Global Trend Data," *Environmental Health Perspectives* 105 (1997): 1228–1232.

5. I. D. Sharlip, et al., "Best Practice Policies for Male Infertility," *Fertility and Sterility* 77, no. 5 (2002): 873–882.

6. J. Lazarou, et al., "Incidence of Adverse Drug Reactions in Hospitalized Patients," *Journal of the American Medical Association* 279, no. 15 (1998): 1200–1205.

7. "Physicians and the Pharmaceutical Industry," *Journal of the American Medical Association* 283, no. 3 (2000).

8. US Consensus Bureau.

9. "Epigenetics," *Nova* (PBS, July 24, 2007) http://www.pbs.org/wgbh/nova/body/epigenetics.html, accessed June, 7, 2016.

CHAPTER 3: PERCEPTION AND ATTITUDE

1. Albert Mehrabian, *Silent Messages*, (Belmont, CA: Wadsworth, 1971).

CHAPTER 4: EMOTIONS

1. "Brain Region Central to Placebo Effect Identified," Eureka Alert, July 18, 2007, http://www.eurekalert.org/pub_releases/2007-07/cp-brc071607.php, accessed June 7, 2016.

CHAPTER 6: RELATIONSHIPS

1. Elizabeth Cohen, "CDC: Antidepressants Most Prescribed Drugs in U.S.," CNN, http://www.cnn.com/2007/HEALTH/07/09/antidepressants/index.html?_s=PM:HEALTH, accessed June 7, 2016.

2. Peter Wehrwein, "Astounding Increase in Antidepressant Use by Americans," Harvard Health Publications, October 20, 2011, www.health.harvard.edu, accessed June 7, 2016.

CHAPTER 8: ALIGNMENT

1. "Forward Head Position," *Mayo Clinic Health Letter* 18, no. 3 (March 2000).

CHAPTER 9: EXERCISE

1. "Exercise and Depression," Harvard Health Publications, June 2009, http://www.health.harvard.edu/mind-and-mood/exercise -and-depression-report-excerpt, accessed June 7, 2016.

CHAPTER 10: REST

1. Institute of Medicine Committee on Sleep Medicine and Research, "Sleep Physiology," Chap. 2 in *Sleep Disorders and Sleep Deprivation: An Unmet Public Health Problem*, by H. Colten and B. Altevogt, eds (2006) http://www.ncbi.nlm.nih.gov/books/ NBK19956/, accessed June 7, 2016.

2. Kulreet Chaudhary, MD, "Sleep and Longevity," *Dr. Oz* (blog), May 27, 2011, http://www.doctoroz.com/blog/kulreet-chaud hary-md/sleep-and-longevity, accessed June 7, 2016.

3. S. L. Woods, E. S. S. Froelicher, S. U. Motzer, and E. Bridges, eds., *Sleep* (Philadelphia: Lippincott Williams and Wilkins, 2005), 197–219.

4. A. Zager, et al., "Effects of Acute and Chronic Sleep Loss on Immune Modulation of Rats," *American Journal of Physiology, Regulatory, Integrative and Comparative Physiology* 293, no. 1 (2007): R504–509.

5. "Napping," National Sleep Foundation, https://sleepfoundation .org/sleep-topics/napping, accessed June 7, 2016.

6. "Snoozing Without Guilt," *Harvard Health Letter*, November 2009, http://www.health.harvard.edu/press_releases/snoozing -without-guilt--a-daytime-nap-can-be-good-for-health, accessed June 7, 2016.

7. "Power Napping for Performance," *The Japan Times*, June 7, 2014, http://www.japantimes.co.jp/opinion/2014/06/07/editorials/ power-napping-performance/#.VfzP2piFOUk, accessed June 7, 2016.

CHAPTER 11: DIET

1. A. P. Simopoulos, L. G. Cleland, eds., "Omega-6/Omega-3 Essential Fatty Acid Ratio: The Scientific Evidence," *World Review of Nutrition and Dietetics* 92 (2003): 1–22.

2. "Why is Dehydration So Dangerous?" Rehydration Project, http://rehydrate.org/dehydration/, accessed June 7, 2016.

3. "The Urinary Tract and How it Works," National Institute of Diabetes and Digestive and Kidney Diseases, http://www .niddk.nih.gov/health-information/health-topics/Anatomy/ urinary-tract-how-it-works/Pages/anatomy.aspx, accessed June 15, 2016.

4. Nutrient Data Laboratory, ARS, USDA National Food and Nutrient Analysis Program.

5. Astaxanthin is a superb natural antioxidant, visit www .algatech.com for more information.

6. Smith and Lowney, PLLC, "The Color Salmon Lawsuit," www .smithandlowney.com/salmon/information, accessed June 7, 2016.

7. Frank B. Hu, et al., "A Prospective Study of Egg Consumption and Risk of Cardiovascular Disease in Men and Women," *The Journal of the American Medical Association* 281, no. 15 (1999).

8. G. M. Shaw, et al., "Periconceptional Dietary Intake of Choline and Betaine and Neural Tube Defects in Offspring," *American Journal of Epidemiology* 160, no. 2 (2004): 102–109.

9. "Farm Animal Welfare: Chickens," The MSPCA-Angell, http://www.mspca.org/programs/animal-protection-legis lation/animal-welfare/farm-animal-welfare/factory-farming/ chicken/chickens-on-the-factory-farm.html, accessed June 15, 2016.

10. "How Pervasive are GMOs in Animal Feed?" GMO Inside, http://gmoinside.org/gmos-in-animal-feed/, accessed June 15, 2016.

11. "Chicken Production on Factory Farms," Farm Sanctuary, http://www.farmsanctuary.org/learn/factory-farming/chickens-used-for-meat/, accessed June 15, 2016.

12. Tabitha Alterman, "Eggciting News!!!" *Mother Earth News*, October 10, 2008 (vitamin D number extrapolated from USDA numbers).

13. USDA Nutrient Database, Whole, Raw Egg, 2007.

14. Cheryl Long and Tabitha Alterman, "Meet Real Free-Range Eggs," *Mother Earth News*, October/November 2007, http://www.motherearthnews.com/real-food/free-range-eggs-zmaz07onzgoe.aspx?PageId=5, accessed August 2016.

15. C. Lu, et al., "Organic Diets Lower Children's Dietary Exposure to Common Agriculture Pesticides," *Environmental Health Perspectives Journal* 113 (2005), http://www.whsc.emory.edu/press_releases_print.cfm?announcement_id_seq=4740, accessed June 7, 2016.

16. F. E. Bear, S. J. Toth, and A. L. Prince, "Variation in Mineral Composition of Vegetables," *Soil Science Society of America Proceedings* 13 (1948): 380–384, http://njaes.rutgers.edu/pubs/bearreport/table4.asp, accessed June 7, 2016.

17. M. Barański, et al., "Higher Antioxidant and Lower Cadmium Concentrations and Lower Incidence of Pesticide Residues in Organically Grown Crops: A Systematic Literature Review and Meta-Analyses," *The British Journal of Nutrition* 112, no. 5 (2014): 1–18.

18. F. Magkos, et al., "Organic Food: Nutritious Food or Food for Thought? A Review of the Evidence," *International Journal of Food Sciences and Nutrition* 54, no. 5 (2003): 357–371.

19. "Food Safety: Frequently Asked Questions About Genetically Modified Foods," World Health Organization, http://www .who.int/foodsafety/areas_work/food-technology/faq -genetically-modified-food/en/, accessed July 10, 2016.

20. Waldon Bello, "Twenty-six Countries Ban GMOs—Why Won't the U.S.?" *The Nation*, October 29, 2013, http://www .thenation.com/article/twenty-six-countries-ban-gmos-why -wont-us/, accessed June 15, 2016.

CHAPTER 12: SUPPLEMENTS

1. National Center for Health Statistics, "Dietary Supplement Use Among U.S. Adults," NCHS Data Brief No. 61 (April 2011), http://www.cdc.gov/nchs/products/databriefs/db61.htm.

2. "Supplement Market Grows to $32.5 Billion," *Nutritional Business Journal*, July 16, 2013, http://newhope.com/research -and-insights/supplement-market-grows-325-billion.

3. Encyclopedia.com, s.v. "Casimir Funk," Encyclopedia.com, http://www.encyclopedia.com/topic/Casimir_Funk.aspx.

4. New York State Office of the Attorney General, "A.G. Schneiderman Asks Major Retailers to Halt Sales of Certain Herbal Supplements," news release, February 3, 2015, http:// www.ag.ny.gov/press-release/ag-schneiderman-asks-major -retailers-halt-sales-certain-herbal-supplements-dna-tests.

5. "Abstracts of the 39th Annual Conference on Cardiovascular Disease Epidemiology and Prevention," *American Heart Association Journal* 99 (1999): 1109–1125.

6. National Institutes of Health, "Vitamin E Fact Sheet for Health Professionals," https://ods.od.nih.gov/factsheets/VitaminE-Health Professional/.

7. S. Budvari, et al., *The Merck Index: An Encyclopedia of Chemicals, Drugs, and Biologicals*, 12th ed. (Whitehouse Station, NJ: Merck Research Laboratories, 1996).

8. National Center for Health Statistics, "Anthropometric Reference Data for Children and Adults, 2007–2010," Weight in Pounds for Women Aged 20 and Over Table 4, Weight in Pounds for Men Aged 20 and Over Table 6, by C. Fryar, et al., http://www.cdc.gov/nchs/data/series/sr_11/sr11_252.pdf.

9. Spalding, et al., "Retrospective Birth Dating of Cells in Humans," *Cell* 122, no. 1 (2005): 133–143.

10. Institute of Medicine Food Forum, "Diet Quality Issues for Aging Adults," presented by K. Tucker in Chap. 5 in *Providing Healthy and Safe Foods as We Age* (2009), http://www.ncbi .nlm.nih.gov/books/NBK51837/#ch5.s1.

CHAPTER 13: INTELLIGENT DESIGN

1. Lee Strobel, *The Case for a Creator: A Journalist Investigates Scientific Evidence That Points to God* (Grand Rapids, MI: Zondervan, 2004), 224.

2. Michael Denton, *Evolution: A Theory in Crisis* (Chevy Chase, MD: Adler & Adler, Publishers, Inc., 1996), 334.

3. Charles Darwin, "Difficulties on Theory," Chap. 6 in *The Origin of Species*, http://www.literature.org/authors/darwin-charles/the -origin-of-species/chapter-06.html, accessed on July 10, 2016.

4. "Science Quotes by Francis Crick," Today in Science History, http://todayinsci.com/C/Crick_Francis/CrickFrancis -Quotations.htm, accessed on July 10, 2016.

5. Yitzhak Paz, et al., "A Submerged Monumental Structure in the Sea of Galilee, Israel," *International Journal of Nautical Archaeology* 42, no. 1 (2013): 189–193.

6. Casey Luskin, "Every Bit Digital: DNA's Programming Really Bugs Some ID Critics," *Salvo Magazine*, March 29, 2010, http://www.discovery.org/a/14391, accessed July 10, 2016.

CHAPTER 14: FAITH

1. "Billy Graham Quotes," AZ Quotes, http://www.azquotes.com/quote/866094, accessed July 10, 2016.

2. R. C. Byrd, "Positive Therapeutic Effects of Intercessory Prayer in a Coronary Care Unit Population." *Southern Medical Journal* 81, no. 7 (1998): 826–829.

3. H. Koenig, "The Relationship Between Religious Activities and Blood Pressure in Older Adults," *The International Journal of Psychology in Medicine* 28, no. 2 (1998): 189–213.

4. Ibid.

5. "How Does Prayer Heal?" *McCall's Magazine*, December 1998.

CHAPTER 15: INPUT/OUTPUT

1. 1910, Edison: His Life and Inventions by Frank Lewis Dyer and Thomas Commerford Martin, Volume 2, Chapter 24: Edison's Method in Inventing, p. 616, Harper & Brothers, New York.

CHAPTER 17: THE 3 EASY STEPS

1. http://newspaperarchive.com/us/indiana/fort-wayne/fort-wayne-sentinel/1902/12-31/page-9.

RESOURCES

Diet

Local farmers markets across all over the world are fantastic options to find local organic produce. That said, American grocery chains like Safeway, Albertsons, Food Lion, Kroger, Publix, Aldi, and others have a "natural" foods offshoot stores or an in-house organic brand. You can also find discounted national organic brands at big box stores like Costco, Sam's and Walmart. Here are some health food-focused grocery chain standouts:

- Whole Foods Market: www.wholefoodsmarket.com
  The clear leader in quality, dependability, selection and innovation in the industry.
- Natural Grocers: www.naturalgrocers.com
  While smaller, they're great and all produce is organic, so you don't have to wonder.
- Sprouts: www.sprouts.com
  Less organic produce, but lots of organic options in all departments and decent prices.
- Trader Joe's: www.traderjoes.com
  80% in-house private label, less organic, but good prices and committed to no GMOs.
- Central Market: www.centralmarket.com and parent company, H-E-B: www.heb .com
  Two Texas powerhouses with a great variety of organic in-house products and produce.
- Harris Teeter: www.harristeeter.com
  A southeast chain with many organic options and healthy eating tools and advice.
- Hannaford: www.hannaford.com
  This northeast chain offers wide variety and healthy eating advice from dieticians.
- PCC Natural Markets: www.pccnaturalmarkets.com
  While only around Seattle, their commitment to non-GMO, organic and local is solid.
- Fairway Market: www.fairwaymarket.com
  All around New York, this growing chain has a good selection of organic products.
- Wheatsville Co-op: www.wheatsville.coop
  A local favorite in Austin since 1976, it's the only retail food co-op in Texas.

Supplements

- Standard Process (SP): www.standardprocess.com
  The oldest whole-food supplement company that still organically grows its raw products.
- MediHerb: www.standardprocess.com/mediherb
  An Australian company with the highest possible quality herbs on the market.
- Garden of Life: www.gardenoflife.com
  An organic whole-food supplement and health food product company.
- Beyond Organic: www.mybeyondorganic.com
  An entire line of natural supplements and health products with a mission.
- Get Real Nutrition: www.getrealnutrition.com
  A completely organic, non-GMO, vegan, gluten free supplement company.
- Juice Plus+: www.juiceplus.com
  While not organic, it is a well-researched whole-food supplement company.

Now, how do you find a good, whole-food nutritionist in your area? Start with your local chiropractor and ask them. Many of them are well-trained. You can also go to the Standard Process website and click on "Health Care Professional Search" under Quick Links or go to: https://www.standardprocess.com/HCP-Search

Alignment

- American Chiropractic Association: www.acatoday.org
- International Chiropractors Association: www.chiropractic.org
- Activator Methods International: www.activator.com
  Find an advanced proficiency rated Activator chiropractor in your area.
- Impulse Adjusting instrument: www.goimpulse.com
  Find a cutting-edge tool-assisted adjustment chiropractor in your area.
- Shannan Chiropractic and Nutrition: www.shannanchiro.com
  My Dad's and my website for our private practice in Austin, Texas.

Exercise

I highly recommend doing an internet search for local classes in Yoga, Pilates, Tai Chi and other full-body fitness programs, and ask a friend where they go, but here is a list of traditional gyms.

- Gold's Gym: www.golds.com
- 24 Hour Fitness: www.24hourfitness.com
- Lifetime Fitness: www.lifetimefitness.com
- Anytime Fitness: www.anytimefitness.com
- Curves Women's Fitness: www.curves.com
- YMCA: www.ymca.net
- Equinox: www.equinox.com

General Health and Nutrition Reading

This is a list of "doctors of the future," authors and books that I find are at least partly on track with the Original Design for Health. As with everything you read, you must decipher if it's right for you.

- Jordan Rubin, NMD, PhD
  Patient Heal Thyself, The Maker's Diet, Perfect Weight America, Planet Heal Thyself
- Andrew Weil, MD
  8 Weeks to Optimum Health, Healthy Aging, True Food, Good Food Fast Food
- William Davis, MD
  Wheat Belly, Wheat Belly: 10-Day Grain Detox
- David Perlmutter, MD
  Grain Brain, Brain Maker
- Amy Myers, MD
  The Autoimmune Solution, The Thyroid Connection
- Don Colbert, MD
  The Seven Pillars of Health, Reversing Inflammation, Let Food Be Your Medicine
- Weston A. Price, DDS
  Nutrition and Physical Degeneration
- Dr. Fab Mancini
  Chicken Soup for the Chiropractic Soul, Feeling Fab, The Power of Self-Healing
- Dr. Mary Enig and Sally Fallon
  Nourishing Traditions, Eat Fat Lose Fat
- Kaayla Daniel, PhD, CCN
  The Whole Soy Story
- Dr. Josh Axe
  Eat Dirt, The Gut Repair Cookbook, The Real Food Diet
- Dr. Pete Sulack
  Unhealthy Anonymous

Spiritual Growth

- Rob Koke
  100 Days of Grace, The Best of the Best
- Dr. Laura Koke
  Wonder, Fit for the King
- Joel Osteen
  Your Best Life Now, I Declare, Fresh Start, Think Better Live Better
- John Eldredge
  Wild at Heart, Beautiful Outlaw, Captivating
- T.D. Jakes
  Let it Go, Woman Thou Art Loosed, He-motions, Destiny, Instinct
- Judah Smith
  Jesus is _____., Life is _____.

Spiritual Growth (continued)

- Rick Warren
  The Purpose Driven Life
- Leon Fontaine
  The Spirit Contemporary Life: Unleashing the Miraculous...
- Don Piper
  Heaven is Real, 90 Minutes in Heaven
- Todd Burpo and Lynn Vincent
  Heaven is for Real: A Little Boy's Astounding Journey...
- Kevin Gerald
  Mind Monsters, Good Things
- Bob George
  Classic Christianity
- Andy Stanley
  Grace

Intelligent Design

- William A. Dembski
  Intelligent Design: The Bridge Between Science & Theology
- Douglas Axe
  Undeniable: How Biology Confirms Our Intuition That Life Is Designed
- Illustra Media: www.illustramedia.com
  Unlocking the Mystery of Life (Movie) & others
- Lee Strobel
  The Case for a Creator
- Michael Denton
  Evolution: Still A Theory in Crisis

Helpful Organizations

- Cornucopia Institute: http://www.cornucopia.org/
  Provides important research and investigations on agricultural and food issues.
- GMO Inside: http://gmoinside.org/
  Provides people with information and tools about genetically modified foods.
- Weston A. Price Foundation: http://www.westonaprice.org/
  Dedicated to restoring nutrient-dense foods to the human diet through education.
- Food Babe: http://foodbabe.com/
  Healthy lifestyle blog and webpage with resources and information.
- The Healthy Home Economist: http://www.thehealthyhomeeconomist.com/
  Website with health news, Real Food recipes, video how-to's about traditional diets.

ABOUT
DR. MARK SHANNAN

Dr. Mark Shannan is a second-generation Chiropractor and Nutritionist, frequent speaker and author who has had a thriving practice in Austin, Texas, for about 20 years. He has a bachelor of science in human anatomy, a doctorate in Chiropractic, and is a certified applied clinical nutritionist. He has an amazing wife and two beautiful daughters who fuel his passion for loving, guiding, and helping others to live the healthiest life achievable.

FREE E-BOOKS?
YES, PLEASE!

Get **FREE** and deeply discounted **Christian books** for your **e-reader** delivered to your inbox **every week!**

IT'S SIMPLE!

VISIT lovetoreadclub.com

SUBSCRIBE by entering your email address

RECEIVE free and discounted e-book offers and inspiring articles delivered to your inbox every week!

Unsubscribe at any time.

SUBSCRIBE NOW!

LOVE TO READ CLUB

visit **LOVETOREADCLUB.COM** ▶

Printed in Great Britain
by Amazon